HOW TO
GET BETTER VALUE
HEALTHCARE

J A MUIR GRAY

First published 2007

Email: books@offoxpress.com
Website: www.offoxpress.com

British Library Cataloguing in Publication Data

Gray, J. A. Muir (John Armstrong Muir)
How to get better value healthcare
   1. Medical care - Great Britain
   I. Title
   362.1'0941

   ISBN-13: 9781904202011

Printed and bound in Great Britain at The Alden Press, De Havilland Way, Witney, OX29 0YG

CONTENTS

A Letter To The Reader

In thirty-five years of managing and paying for healthcare, I have made all the mistakes, most of them only once. In *How To Get Better Value Healthcare* I have attempted to set out the methods I have used to get better value in jobs which have covered every type of care from ante-natal to terminal, and which have had responsibility for budgets ranging from a billion a year to zero, the latter actually offering surprising opportunities. When it is impossible to invest more money, people have to change, and in the words of Cool Hand Luke, 'sometimes nothing is the coolest hand.'

My experience has been solely in the public sector but these methods will all be relevant in the independent sector. Those who pay for or manage private sector healthcare do, of course, face pressures unknown in the public sector, but there are two pressures they do not feel – firstly those which come from the need to deliver healthcare for a whole population and secondly those which come from a fixed budget. These constraints have, however, created an intellectual framework for decision-making which suited my aim – the promotion of evidence-based decision-making.

More than twenty years ago we started training people who manage healthcare in what we called 'applied epidemiology'. The training was based on the hypothesis that clinical epidemiology was a core skill for those who pay for or manage healthcare, a 'contextual skill' of relevance only to healthcare, to complement 'general management skills', such as leadership, of relevance in all organisations.

Kindred spirits were encountered at McMaster University, and their book entitled *Clinical Epidemiology – a Basic Science* (1) was inspirational. In Oxford, we were stimulated by the arrival of one of McMaster's luminaries, Dave Sackett, and the happy precipitation of a number of individuals and organisations interested primarily in the quality of knowledge rather than the quantity; the influence of the Cochrane Collaboration's presence was immense, and Iain Chalmers continues to provide me with advice and stimulation. From this minestrone emerged evidence-based healthcare, the use of best current evidence in making decisions about groups of patients or populations complemented by two other elements – the needs and the values of the population.

Evidence-based decision-making is rational but, having worked in the public sector, often in the public eye, the emotional and ethical aspects of decision-making have always been prominent. Healthcare decisions should be based on rational economic evidence, but decision-making in what Herbert Simon calls the 'buzzing blooming confusion' that constitutes the real world requires the judgement to combine rational and non-rational decisions to make a 'good enough' decision in imperfect conditions. Very rarely is a decision-maker choosing whether or not to fund a new treatment or service from a fund just waiting to be spent; usually the decision-makers face a multitude of problems and options. They have only a small amount of high quality information, the evidence, about how the intervention has worked in a research setting, and a great deal of low quality information and uncertainty about the effect of the intervention in their service. The 'fog of war' is the famous Clausewitz phrase, describing decision-making in war, perhaps the closest analogy to decision-making in healthcare. In healthcare, as in war, decisions have to be made. Every decision means that some patients will do better, others will suffer. These are hellish decisions from which there is no escape, and this book has been written to help those who have to make them.

J. A. Muir Gray

Reference

(1) Sackett, D.L., Haynes, R.B., Guyatt, G.H., Tugwell, P. (1991) Clinical Epidemiology – A Basic Science. *Lippincot Williams & Wilkins*

PART I

THE 21ST CENTURY HEALTHCARE CRISIS

Chapter 1

THE MEANINGS OF VALUE

ONE OPERATION: FOUR PERSPECTIVES

'Oh fuck!' said the surgeon, gazing at the liver newly exposed by his generous incision from the sternum to the umbilicus.

Human liver looks like calves' liver or lamb's liver – smooth, firm, shiny, and cerise. The human liver is a large organ. It lies just below the rib cage with a large lobe on the right side tapering to a left lobe which lies across the midline. The liver is a generous organ. It has more capacity than is needed and good health is possible even if half the liver is destroyed or removed. The liver is a bloody organ. The large amount of blood that flows through the liver means that cancer cells often lodge and grow in the liver to become metastases or secondaries, and these 'liver secondaries' were regarded as a death sentence until advances in surgery and anaesthesia enabled surgical treatment, and perhaps cure, if the secondaries were situated in the left lobe of the liver which can be detached from the right main lobe and removed.

Ten days before surgery, x-rays had found secondaries only in the left lobe of the liver, but when the liver lay exposed under the merciless theatre lights, little white specks covered the surface of the right lobe and the left lobe; surgical treatment would therefore be futile.

'Oh, fuck!' said the surgeon and, after a pause, 'Let's go ahead anyway.'

The trainee's perspective

That Catholics enjoyed themselves on Sundays was a cause of universal disapproval to Scottish Presbyterians in the nineteen-seventies, and a cause of envy to not a few. After Mass, Catholics could relax and enjoy themselves, although in a Scottish city in those days the opportunities for enjoyment on the Sabbath were few. The young doctor, who had spent seven hours on the liver operation, and kept watch in the evening on the patient's post-operative course, received no extra pay. There was no direct cost to him, but, even in Scotland, he could have spent the day going to church, playing golf, sleeping, or studying.

The opportunity cost was high but he regarded it as negligible, both at the time and in retrospect, because his frustration at this experience was one of the reasons that he decided to leave surgery, a move of great value to himself and to those future patients who would have undeniably received poor quality care from an academic surgeon whose strengths and weaknesses were better suited to a career in public health.

The payer's and manager's perspective

The perspective of the hospital management and the payer, the local NHS Board, are not recorded because they never knew the operation was taking place. The theatre that was used was available for emergencies and some direct costs were entailed, swabs and sutures, for example, but the staff would have spent the day on cleaning and maintenance, or reading the ubiquitous *Sunday Post*, had the operation not appeared on the theatre list; no other operation had to be postponed or delayed as a consequence.

Had they known it was happening, the manager and the payer might have viewed it as a worthwhile investment, although it is to be hoped that they would have classified it as a futile investment of resources had they appreciated the significance of the secondaries in the right-hand lobe of the liver. If the right-hand lobe of the liver had been clear of secondaries, the operation, the first of its kind in that hospital, would almost certainly have been classified as progress, and progress has both cost and value.

The development of new skills within a hospital or health service not only allows it to improve the health of the population it serves but also allows it to attract more patients, increase the hospital income, and allow further capital investment and staff recruitment.

The surgeon's perspective

From the surgeon's perspective, the operation was valuable. The exposure and ligation of the left hepatic artery and vein, the preservation of the common bile duct, and the satisfactory sealing of the large exposed surface of the liver from which the left lobe had been sliced off, had all gone well. The condition of the patient was satisfactory during and after surgery. The presence of the secondaries in the right lobe was to be regretted. The operation was not curative but others would be: the surgeon had now done a hemi-hepatectomy. This operation is now a standard operation and he, like other surgeons, performed many of them with success, but progress has to start somewhere. There has to be a first patient to be given penicillin or have a heart transplant, and for each surgeon there has to be a first – and the price can be high.

In a brave series of papers, a respected cardiac surgeon reported how mortality increased temporarily when he changed his technique before falling to levels much lower than with his old technique. Progress has a price as well as a reward.

The patient's perspective

The perspective of the patient although not on record, would depend both upon what she was told, and her personal values. She probably valued the operation highly, because many patients appreciate the fact that their clinicians are trying everything that can be done to beat cancer. Even if she had been told that there were secondaries left behind, at least some had been cut out, and for some patients that would have been of high value. It may have been that the secondaries left in the right lobe would have lain quiet for years. Such a possibility, remote though it is, cannot be dismissed.

The word 'value' has, like many words, more than one meaning. One meaning is a statement of principle, for example 'respect for the autonomy of the individual patient is one of our core values'. Economists use the word in a different way. They talk about the value that investment in healthcare produces, which is the difference between the good that the service does and the harm that it does in proportion to the amount of resources used. Although the term 'value' has the same general meaning for payers, patients, clinicians and managers, and for the industries that produce drugs, equipment and IT for them, all four use it in different ways.

MULTIPLE MEANINGS AND DEFINITIONS

The payer's value

From the perspective of payers for healthcare, whose responsibility it is to allocate money among different groups of patients, and, if the government is the payer, different jurisdictions, value is at its maximum when it is impossible to increase the good, or decrease the harm, by reallocating a single pound or euro from one group of patients to another, or from one part of the country to another.

The patient's value

From the perspective of the patient, the value of the care received is measured not just by the outcome of the care they receive, but by the way it is delivered.

The value that patients place on the service they have received will be reduced if, for example, they feel that:

- their time has been wasted waiting in a clinic for a consultation in which laboratory results were unavailable
- they were treated rudely and impersonally
- they did not receive as much information as they wished

Even if the patient is not paying directly, their valuation of the service is of central importance. Good outcomes are necessary but not sufficient; good patient experience will also be of essential importance to the 21st century patient, and therefore to those who provide and pay for their care.

The clinician's value

Busy clinicians highly value the opportunity to use their time, their scarcest resource, to see those patients most likely to benefit from their skill, and to provide for each patient the best care that patient needs quickly and easily. Most clinicians now accept that 'best' means the best that can be provided by the service in which they are working. This may be different from everything that is possible for a particular patient were costs not a consideration. The clinician in a world in which resources were limitless might try treatments which could give hope, and which might work for one in a million patients. However, when working in a system in which payers have to derive maximum value for the whole population for which they are responsible, treatments with this level of benefit – the offer of hope combined with a one in a million chance of success – is of too low a value to be acceptable, and would therefore not be included in the range of treatment options available to the clinician working in the service. Not all clinicians find this tension easy to bear.

The manager's value

The meaning of 'value' to a manager is akin to that of the payer because managers are responsible for groups of patients, not individuals. They want the care to be effective and safe for the individual in order to minimise complaints, which are time-consuming and bad for morale, and errors, which can be expensive for the organisation. But most of all, the manager wants productivity.

The manager of a healthcare facility such as a hospital is rarely told by the payer how much to invest for each patient group. She may be told to invest in a service where there are obvious deficiencies, usually manifest by long waiting times. A manager has to allocate resources into three main types of spend – direct clinical care, clinical support services such as biochemistry, and management.

The management team of a health service also has to decide which services should get more money, or, in times of retrenchment, which should get less. The manager of a health service values most her ability to deliver care of a standard that will maximise the possibility of benefit and minimise the possibility of harm, while satisfying their payers' requirements and continuously improving their service. The scarcest resource for a manager is freedom of action.

Industry's value

Although it is common to talk about the healthcare industry, healthcare is a service which does, however, stimulate and support pharmaceutical, equipment, diagnostic and IT industries.

Frequently industrial developers of new products or services are disappointed by the lack of enthusiasm generated by their latest product or service. The reason for this is not simply the added cost that the new technology will require, at least in the short term, but the failure to appreciate the different meanings of the term 'value', complicated by the fact that many health services are so hard-pressed financially that they are unable to create a fund, sometimes called an 'invest-to-save' fund, that would allow the necessary investment in the short term to increase value in the long term.

Dictionary definitions of value

There are two types of dictionary. Those which give only the definition of the lexicographer who wrote it, like Dr Johnson's dictionary. The second type of dictionary, requiring massively more resources, at a level not available to Dr Johnson, gives not only the lexicographer's definition but also examples of the word in use. For instance, the *Shorter English Dictionary* clearly distinguishes between two different meanings of the word 'value', both in common use in healthcare.

One meaning of the word value may be described as its moral meaning, namely 'the status of a thing or the estimate in which it is held according to its real or supposed worth, usefulness, or importance', the definition from the late Middle English. This use of the word 'value' is common in healthcare, for example the hospital which claims that 'we value patient choice', or 'we value openness and honesty'.

The second meaning in the Shorter English Dictionary can be described as the economic meaning, and one of the four variants that the Shorter English Dictionary gives is 'that amount of some commodity, medium of exchange, etc. which is considered to be an equivalent for something else', and it gives as an example of the meaning of the term the use in 1806 'we could hardly be said to have value for our money'. In the specialised *Healthcare Economics Dictionary*, published by Anthony Culyer in 2005 (1), the author, acting as lexicographer, defines value by saying that 'in economics, value is usually taken as a maximum amount that an individual or group is willing to pay for a particular good or service rather than go without it.' He also defines 'marginal value' as 'the value of marginal benefit: the maximum an individual is willing to pay for an increment of benefit'.

On 24 June 2006, Wikipedia, which calls itself an encyclopaedia but also acts as a dictionary, provided eight different meanings of the word 'value'. One of these is the meaning that is used in this book:

'value (economics)'. In an excellent one-liner, Wikipedia states that 'in general, the value of something is how much a product or service is worth to someone, relative to other things (often measured in money)'.

The word 'value' is now widely used in medical literature, but if one searches for value one finds articles which relate not only to words but also, mercifully, to numbers.

Numerical definitions of value

The Vienna School of Philosophy flourished in the 1920s and 1930s and became very influential in Britain, where it gave rise to what is known as 'logical positivism'. Their leading light in Britain was A. J. Ayer, whose book *Language, Truth and Logic* (2), published in 1935 when he was twenty-four, had a massive impact. The logical positivists took an approach to definition of the meaning of a term that did not rely on words alone. In his book, Ayer said that:

> *'Instead of trying to understand the meaning of a proposition by analysing the meaning of the individual words that compose it, another approach should be taken. The criterion which we use to test the genuineness of apparent statements of facts is the criterion of verifiability. We say that a sentence is factually significant to any given person if, and only if, he knows how to verify the proposition which it purports to express – that is, if he knows what observations will lead him, under certain conditions, to accept the proposition as being true, or reject it as being false. And with regard to questions, the procedure is the same. We enquire in every case what observations will lead us to answer the question one way or the other, and, if none can be discovered, we must conclude that the sentence under consideration does not, as far as we are concerned, express a genuine question, however strongly its grammatical appearance may suggest that it does.'*

An example of numerical expressions of value which would please A. J. Ayer is set out below.

> *'Alternating pressure mattresses were associated with lower overall costs (£283.06 per patient on average, 95% confidence interval £377.59 to £976.79) mainly due to*

reduced lengths of stay in hospital and greater benefits (a delay in time to ulceration of 10.64 days on average, 24.40 to 3.09)' (3)

For many years, the benefits of healthcare interventions were measured in terms of the numbers of years of life added. The use of the number of years of life gained as the criterion used to assess new, or existing, healthcare interventions led to a focus on length of life as the aim of healthcare, with priority being given to research on, and subsequent investment in services for, 'killer diseases'.

People who had, or people who looked after people who had, chronic disabling diseases that did not significantly affect the length of life, such as depression, argued that this approach discriminated against disabling diseases, and as a consequence steps were taken to develop measurements that would take into account quality of life as well as quantity.

A key paper was published in 1978 by Rosser and Kind called *A Scale of Valuations of States of Illness: Is There a Social Consensus?* (4). This paper was of immense importance and led to the development of a measure called the quality adjusted life year (QALY), which is a measure of health-related quality of life, taking into account both quantity and quality. A year of perfect health was deemed to be worth 1, death was usually given 0, although society agrees that there are some situations that could be regarded as worse than death and which need negative numbers. Although there has been much debate about the QALY, it is still the least worst measure that can be used to assess the value of a particular intervention.

The development of the Disability Adjusted Life Year has also been of great importance for policy-makers, and in the 1996 publication *The Global Burden of Disease* (5), the World Health Organisation included quality adjusted measures as well as mortality in a significant review of previous thinking on healthcare priorities. This major work, edited by Murray and Lopez, significantly changed the ranking of diseases and brought mental health problems much higher up the league table of human suffering.

REACHING AGREEMENT ON MEANING

Because there are multiple meanings and definitions, it is essential to reach agreement on how the term 'meaning' will be used.

In *How To Get Better Value Healthcare*, the term will be used to mean 'the net health benefit, that is the difference between the benefit and the harm done by a service, taking into account the amount of resources invested.'

In every meeting in which value is to be discussed, either implicitly or explicitly, it is essential to reach agreement on a single meaning that can be used - if only for the duration of the meeting. How to do that is described in Part III of this book.

References

(1) Culyer, A. (2005) Healthcare Economics Dictionary. *Cheltenham: Edward Elgar*
(2) Ayer, A.J. (1935) Language, Truth and Logic. *Penguin*
(3) Iglesias et al (2006) Pressure Relieving Support Surfaces (PRESSURE) Trial: Cost-effectiveness Analysis. *BMJ 332: 1416-1418*
(4) Rosser, R. & Kind, P. (1978) A Scale of Valuations of States of Illness: Is there a Social Consensus? *Internat. J. Epidemiol. 7: 347-358.*
(5) Murray, C.J.L. & Lopez, A.D. (1996) The Global Burden of Disease. *WHO*, Geneva

Chapter 2

THE CHALLENGES OF 21st CENTURY HEALTHCARE

INCREASING NEED

Twentieth century healthcare was dominated by clinicians, effectiveness, and efficiency. Twenty first century healthcare will be dominated by patients and value, because the challenges facing 21st century healthcare in every society are massive, and growing. All developed countries are putting more resources into healthcare, but in every country the increase in financial investment is insufficient to meet the remorseless increase in need and demand (Figure 2.1).

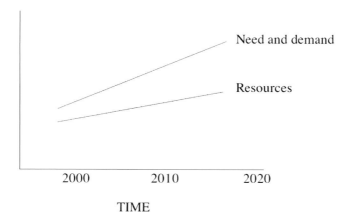

TIME

Figure 2.1 *The widening gap between resources and need*

Furthermore, even if more money could be made available, the human resources might not be forthcoming. As societies become richer, fewer people are willing to carry out the basic tasks, often aesthetically unsavoury, involved in caring for sick people. As a result many developed countries have taken to plundering the human resources of poorer countries, employing a significant proportion of the medical and nursing graduates from poor countries. Fortunately, many countries now regard this as something which is undesirable, whereas formerly it was accepted as an economic necessity. Even if recruitment were to continue, however, the basic premise remains the same and is demonstrated in Figure 2.1. Need and demand are increasing faster than the resources available to meet them.

There are three inter-related contributors to increasing need, illustrated below (Figure 2.2).

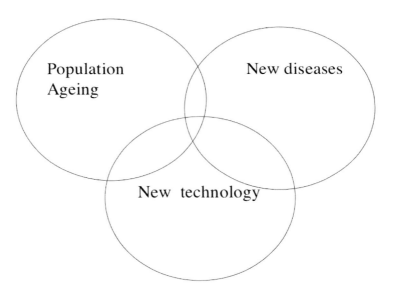

Figure 2.2 *The causes of increasing need*

Population ageing

In almost every society, the number of people aged over 80 is increasing dramatically. The main reason for this trend is not that the death rate of people in their seventies is declining dramatically as a result of better medical care; it is because the percentage of children who survived the perilous years of infancy rose significantly seven decades ago.

There is good evidence that people aged over eighty are fitter now than people aged over eighty were twenty or thirty years ago. However, even fitter old people have a higher prevalence of chronic disease, so the number of people suffering from chronic diseases increases as a result of population aging. In addition, whether people die at 70, 80, or 90 years of age, the last few months of life is a time in which there is usually heavy use of health services. An increase in the number of people surviving to old age inevitably increases the need.

New disease

Twenty-first century healthcare has to cope not only with the diseases it inherited from the 20th century but also with new diseases. Indeed, in many poor countries, health services have still to cope not only with the 19th century epidemics of tuberculosis, cholera, and infant malnutrition, but also with heart disease and road traffic accidents. In developed countries, health services have to cope with the problems that have evolved in the 20th century as a consequence of lifestyle changes and population ageing. However, the list is not closed.

The last decade has seen the emergence of AIDS, SARS and Avian flu, and the evolution of epidemics of problems in which social changes, the media, and some clinicians, have led to epidemics of new conditions such as anorexia nervosa, false memory syndrome, and ME. The evolution of these epidemics, each a real problem for the affected individual, is acutely analysed in *Hystories* by Elaine Showalter. (1)

The Venn diagram in Figure 2.2 shows that these drivers are inter-related, for example:

- Some of the new technology reduces the risk of surgical intervention and allows older people who would not have been considered fit for operation in the past to be treated; this also increases the need for healthcare.
- Attitudes are different. Now neither older people nor clinicians are willing to accept health problems as being caused by 'old age', and rightly so. The expectation of both is that people with health problems who ask for help should have the same opportunity for diagnosis and treatment, whatever their age. This increases the demand for healthcare.

New technology

A useful definition of a health need is a health problem for which there is an effective intervention. For this reason, when a new drug or other type of medical technology is invented and approved for use, a new need is also created.

MANAGING NEED

There is very little that those who pay for or manage healthcare can do to slow the increase in need. If those who pay for healthcare are also responsible for the public health, they need to do what they can to prevent the epidemics of smoking-related diseases, or diseases related to addiction, and the consequences of obesity, for each of these will have a massive impact on healthcare. If the payers for healthcare do not have responsibilities for public health, all they can do is hope that those who do will take effective action, because there is no other action to prevent the increase in disease. Population ageing is a given fact, determined in part by the effectiveness of modern healthcare but determined much more by the fall in infant mortality six or seven decades ago. Governments can attempt to control the growth of new technology by refusing to fund research and development, but that would have little effect because the major funder of new technology is now industry, not government.

All that those who pay for, or manage, healthcare can do is to manage the introduction of new technology and promote the extinction of redundant technology to ensure that maximum value is derived from resources invested.

INCREASING DEMAND

The demand for healthcare is also increasing as a result of a general trend call consumerism, fuelled by the Internet. The demand for healthcare is not easily managed. Various options are possible, one of which is to be explicit about healthcare conditions which will or will not be given treatment from publicly funded health services. These might include gender reassignment operations, symptomless inguinal hernia, aesthetic surgery, symptomless varicose veins, and symptomless gallstones.

In addition, services may make explicit the decisions not to fund interventions which they deem to be of low value, such as bariatric surgery for obesity, intensive in-patient treatment for addiction, and operative repair of cruciate ligaments of the knee except for active sportsmen and women.

A strong case can be made on the grounds of effectiveness for all these treatments, but management of demand is not possible if left to individual clinicians faced with the distress of the individual patient, and funders have to make decisions at a population level.

Managing demand

Managing demand is not easy but some steps can be taken, for example:

- be very clear and explicit about the sub-groups of patients most likely to benefit from an intervention and, as a corollary, those who are least likely to benefit;
- express the probability of benefit in absolute terms rather than relative terms, because the use of absolute rather than relative risk communication of benefits and harms almost always reduces the demand for care. For this reason evangelists for a new service usually express the benefits in relative rather than absolute terms, to gain an effect known as 'framing';
- ensure that patients are given information about the risks and limitations of intervention as well as the benefits;
- provide full information for patients in different media, for example by the use of patient reports about failed treatment as well as data.

These steps can be incorporated into patient decision aids, part of an effective patient engagement strategy. (2) One of the effects of widespread diffusion of the view of medical progress, influenced strongly by what has been called 'optimism bias', is that the public are keen for treatment. One of the benefits of promoting evidence-based patient choice in which patients are given high quality information about benefits, risks and limitations, to counteract optimism bias, is to reduce demand.

Managing clinical demand

'There is a fashion in operations, as there is in sleeves and skirts: the triumph of some surgeon who has at last found out how to make a once desperate operation fairly safe is usually followed by a rage for that operation not only among the doctors, but actually among their patients.'
George Bernard Shaw (1906), Preface to 'The Doctor's Dilemma'

Demand is generated as often by clinicians as by patients. In its most overt form, clinician enthusiasm can contribute to the development of epidemics such as the false memory syndrome, but an enthusiastic medical profession, altruistic and keen to do good, armed with information provided by enthusiastic promoters of new technology, expressed in terms of relative benefit rather than absolute benefit are, not surprisingly, the people who fuel the growth in demand. Clinical demand may be overtly expressed, for example by clinicians leading a campaign for a new service or a new facility such as a PET scanner.

Sometimes, science may be put into practice by a well-considered national policy decision – for example, the introduction in the UK of breast cancer screening. However, many innovations are introduced into clinical practice by clinicians, who then seek the resources to fund the innovation from those who pay for the service to be delivered. The ways in which changes or innovations in clinical practice increase the cost of care are manifold (see Table 2.1).

A study by Eddy in the USA (4) showed that, in a healthcare system in which expenditure is not finite, changes in the 'volume and intensity' of clinical practice are the main factors driving increases in the cost of care that can be controlled by health service managers. The other causes of increasing costs – population ageing, medical and general price inflation – are beyond the power of health service managers to control (Figure 2.3, page 17).

In other healthcare systems in which decisions are made within a context of finite resources, although expenditure does not spiral out of control, changes in the volume and intensity of clinical practice will generate financial and service pressures and can also drive the service in directions other than those that have been identified as priorities, for instance those on the new management agenda.

Managing innovation usually focuses on a small number of potentially high-cost interventions, for example the number of MRI

Table 2.1: How Innovations In Clinical Practice Increase Costs

- Treating conditions that were previously untreatable.

- Treating people who would previously have been untreated because of changing professional perceptions of need and appropriateness and changing public expectations. These may result from:

  ○ Increasing safety of intervention;
  ○ More acceptable, less invasive, more pleasant interventions;
  ○ Changing attitudes to chronological age as a reason for refusing treatment;
  ○ Changing expectations about health and disease.

- Providing more expensive types of treatment:

  ○ More expensive drugs;
  ○ More expensive imaging;
  ○ More expensive tests;
  ○ More expensive staff.

- More intensive clinical practice:

  ○ Longer duration of stay;
  ○ More tests per patient;
  ○ More professional interventions per patient;
  ○ More treatments per patient.

Source: Evidence-Based Healthcare (3)

---

machines. However, the conclusion from David Eddy's work, which is as true today as when it was published, is that every innovation, no matter how small, needs to have its introduction to, or removal from, the healthcare system carefully managed, particularly if it is for a common disease. The proposal that a screening test be introduced to the adult population would mean that even if the test cost only £1 to administer, the total cost in the UK would be about £20 million. Even

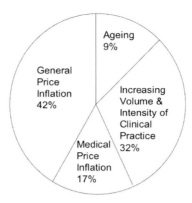

Figure 2.3 *The causes of cost inflation*

the administrative consequences of a simple test could amount to £10 million, and if a percentage of the population required further investigation the further bill for a simple procedure can easily enter the hundreds of millions, even if there is no clear evidence of added value.

References

(1) Showalter, E. (1997) Hystories: Hysterical Epidemics and Modern Culture. *Columbia Univ. Press*

(2) Gray, J.A.M. (2005) The Resourceful Patient. *eRosetta Press*

(3) Gray, J.A.M. (2002) Evidence-Based Healthcare. *Elsevier*

(4) Eddy, D.M. (1993) Three Battles to Watch in the 1990s. *JAMA 270: 520-526*

Chapter 3

THE BEST RESPONSE TO 21st CENTURY CHALLENGES

ARCHIE COCHRANE'S 'RANDOM REFLECTIONS'

In the last three decades of the 20th century, health service payers and managers were appropriately preoccupied with effectiveness and efficiency, and only services that did more good than harm at reasonable cost were considered for funding.

However, of developed countries, only the United Kingdom faced serious resource constraints in the 1980s and was forced to think about opportunity costs rather than simply taking new interventions which had a favourable result from cost-benefit or cost-effectiveness analysis. Since then, every other major developed economy, which is committed to offering healthcare to its whole population, has had to face up to limits placed on healthcare spending. In Germany, Japan, and Italy for example, evidence-based decision-making has become much more explicit. The United States remains an exception. There is certainly concern about healthcare costs in many sectors of American society, but insurance companies will provide cover for any service that their members, or their employers, will pay for, and within each insurance company or health maintenance organisation, fierce debates take place. The United States as a whole, however, does not have this debate because there is not a national commitment to cover the whole population. It was in the United Kingdom, therefore, that the response to the work of Archie Cochrane was most enthusiastic.

> 'He lived and died, a severe porphyric, who smoked too much, without the consolation of a wife, a religious belief, or a merit award, but he didn't do too badly.'

These were the words chosen by Archie Cochrane when he wrote his own biography for the *British Medical Journal*. As befits the man, they were ironic, clear, accurate, and understated. Few people have had more influence on healthcare in the last fifty years of the 20th century than Archie Cochrane, firstly by his insistence on the importance of the randomised controlled trial, secondly by his challenge to the medical and research establishments that they should organise all of their knowledge properly, leading to the creation of the Cochrane Collaboration, and thirdly by the publication of his *Random Reflections on Health Services* in 1972, with the title *Effectiveness and Efficiency* (1). This small book was published and the aim of 20th century healthcare became effectiveness and efficiency.

EFFECTIVENESS: A KEY 20th CENTURY CONCEPT

'All effective treatments must be free.' This, wrote Cochrane, was the device his banner carried at a Communist rally in the 1930s, written after considerable thought but making no impact on the communists on the march. But it did make an impact on Cochrane, who remained obsessed with the need for treatments to be demonstrated to be effective and then, if they were, for those treatments to be made available through a National Health Service. For Cochrane it was clear that the single best method for demonstrating the effectiveness of a treatment was the randomised controlled clinical trial, and he promoted the importance of the trial with commitment, energy, intelligence, and a considerable degree of cunning throughout the rest of his professional career. As a result the term 'effectiveness' entered the general vocabulary, not only of the research worker but of all those who manage and pay for healthcare.

Cochrane, however, not only promoted effectiveness. He also wrote of the need for efficiency; it is worthwhile considering how he used the term 'efficiency', and the best means of doing this is a quote from his *Random Reflections*.

> *'There are two preliminary steps which are essential before this cost/benefit approach becomes a practical possibility and it is with these two steps that I am chiefly concerned. The first is, of course, to measure the effect of a particular medical action in altering the natural history of a particular*

disease for the better. Since the introduction of the randomized controlled trial (RCT) our knowledge in this sphere has greatly increased but is still sadly limited. It is in this sense I use the word 'effective' in this book, and I use it in relation to research results, as opposed to the results obtained when a therapy is applied in ordinary clinical practice in a defined community. Some people would like to use the word 'efficacious' for this measurement. This seems reasonable, but as I do not like the word I have not used it here.'

After thirty-five years in common use, the term 'effective', inevitably, is now used much more loosely, and has many different meanings. Some people still use it with the original meaning. For many clinicians, however, 'effective' is used to mean that, in their experience, patients appear to have got better, or even that a single patient had got better while using the treatment.

Defining ineffectiveness

The people who argued most strongly for the need for Cochrane's definition of effectiveness to be adopted also pointed out that 'absence of evidence of effectiveness is not proof of absence of effect'. This allows people to argue that the absence of evidence of effect in, for example, breast cancer screening in women under the age of 50, was simply due to the fact that the trials that had been organised were too small, and that the proposition that 'screening for breast cancer in women under 50 is ineffective' was simply a statement of effectiveness according to the rules laid down by those who funded research and healthcare. There is some truth in this accusation.

Another reason why the term 'effective' fell into disrepute was that treatments have both good and bad effects, but the word 'effective' had come to be synonymous with good effects, reflecting in part the problems of positive publication bias. This has encouraged researchers and editors to publish articles describing the positive effects of new treatments but ignoring the potential harms of treatments, a phenomenon known as optimism bias. (2)

The limitations of 'effectiveness'

For these reasons, the term 'effective' is no longer useful as a means of sharply distinguishing 'the effective' from 'the ineffective' Instead of the shorthand term 'effective', therefore, it has become common to talk about the balance between good and harm, for example by describing the results of research in terms of both benefits and harms. Some interventions, such as prostate cancer screening, have weak evidence of benefit and strong evidence of harm, whereas other treatments, such as Statins, have strong evidence of considerable benefit with strong evidence that harm is uncommon. Furthermore, we are far beyond the era in which 'all effective treatments must be free', and in every society there are examples of 'effective' treatments, if we wish to continue using that term, which cannot be afforded for the whole population.

It is certainly necessary to demonstrate that a new intervention, screening, diagnostic test, or treatment, does more good than harm by good quality research, preferably by a systematic review of all existing research, but that by itself is no longer a guarantee of funding. In an attempt to resolve this problem, governments and payers have had increasingly to turn to Archie Cochrane's second great legacy – efficiency – as the criterion by which interventions should be judged.

'EFFICIENCY' – A KEY 20th CENTURY CONCEPT

The multiple meanings of the term 'efficiency' illustrate Wittgenstein's principle that arguments result from a failure of the parties concerned to agree on the meaning of the terms they are using. (3) Two people can have a furious argument about whether or not a health service is efficient, when one is in fact talking about cost-effectiveness and the other about productivity – two of the commonly used definitions of efficiency.

The productivity of a health service relates the inputs to the outputs, for example the number of cases per bed or the number of operations per surgeon. The efficiency or cost-effectiveness relates the outcomes to inputs, for example the number of people cured related to the operations carried out.

The term 'productivity' was defined by Anthony Culyer as 'the output of goods and services produced by one or more factors of production'. (4) For him, 'a factor of production' is synonymous with input, and is now widely used without reference to efficiency. For example, in a *British Medical Journal* editorial on 'Healthcare productivity', the authors do not use the term efficiency, even though they are concerned with outcomes rather than outputs. (5)

The limitations of 'efficiency'

The use of quality adjusted life years allows the cost and benefit of different services to be expressed in the same currency and this in turn allows services to be compared with both one another and with some threshold above which services are not regarded as 'cost-effective'. This approach has been very helpful and has been widely used, notably by NICE in the United Kingdom and by the Australian Drugs Reimbursement Committee. (6, 7)

However, even the use of this criterion does not solve all the problems of decision makers, principally because most societies are now faced with the prospect of having more interventions which come within the threshold of cost-effectiveness than can be afforded by health services. As with effectiveness, efficiency is necessary but not sufficient. It is certainly important for every society to adopt some means of appraising the costs and benefits of interventions that clinicians or industry offer to them, but this will not solve all the problems, in part because of having more interventions that meet the criteria than can be afforded, in part because people with rare diseases may present very challenging problems to decision-makers.

The treatment a person with a rare disease requires often falls outside the threshold of cost-effectiveness but, if not funded, will result in the death of an individual, sometimes an individual whose name and image has become familiar to the public and to politicians. This is something society finds difficult to accept.

OPTIMALITY AS A 21st CENTURY CONCEPT

Avedis Donabedian was an Armenian, and his nationality was in many ways as important to him as were Cochrane's roots in Scotland. In 2003, Oxford University Press published a book whose copyright rested with the American University of Armenia entitled *An Introduction to Quality Assurance in Health Care*. (8) In his preface, Donabedian states that: 'It was with great reluctance that I undertook to write this book', but from 'the happy state' of his retirement, he felt he was recalled by 'the urgent need, insistently and repeatedly brought to my attention, for a brief, coherent account of quality assurance in health care for use by students of the subject in my native Armenia'.

Donabedian wrote the book during the end stages of what his editor describes as 'combat with an avaricious cancer that weakened his musculature but left his mind untouched', and the book was published in the year 2000, three years after his death at the age of 81. The book is outstanding, only 200 pages long, but pulling together a lifetime's work of clear thinking. Donabedian's previous classic was his three volume Explorations in Quality Assessment and Monitoring, published in 1980 (9), and it was in this work that he described not only structure, process, and outcome but also his 'unifying model of benefit, risk and cost'. The power of this model is that it described for the first time the fact that as resources are increased in healthcare, benefit increases, but the increase in benefit then flattens off, illustrating what some people have called the Law of Diminishing Returns (Figure 3.1).

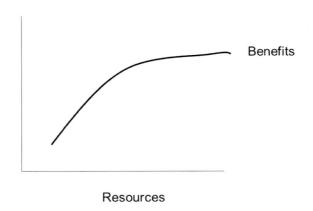

Resources

Figure 3.1 *The Law of Diminishing Benefit*

In contrast, the amount of harm done increases in direct proportion to the investment of resources. For each unit of increase in resource, there is a unit increase in the volume of care, and a unit increase in the amount of harm. In fact there may be a progressive increase in the amount of harm if, with each unit of increase in the availability of care, patients who are less fit and more at risk of harm are covered by the service (Figure 3.2).

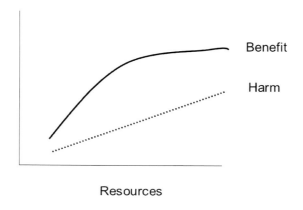

Figure 3.2 *The Law of Undiminishing Harm*

As a consequence, there may come a point where the investment of additional resources will lead to a reduction in the net benefit, calculated by subtracting the harm from the benefit. This is sometimes called the 'health gain'. Donabedian's prose is crystal clear:

> *'If benefits to health are used as the sole criterion of quality, there is no clear-cut level of service which corresponds to optimum care. One must presumably continue to add services until no measurable additional benefits accrue, but that is to proceed without considering the risk that is inherent to a greater or lesser degree in all health care...the services prescribe the use first of large benefits and small risk. Then, as services are added, each increment has progressively larger risks and smaller benefits...the curve of 'benefits against risks' rises to a peak.'*

In his last book, Donabedian describes optimality explicitly as:

> *'The balancing of improvements in health against the cost of such improvements. The definition implies there is a 'best' or 'optimum relationship' between costs and benefits of health care, a point below which more benefits could be obtained at costs that are low relative to benefits and above which additional benefits are obtained at costs too large relative to corresponding benefits.' (Figure 3.3)*

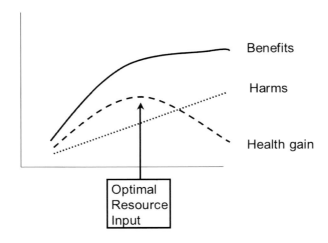

Figure 3.3 *The optimal relationship between resources, benefit and harm*

Clinicians and patient groups often desire maximally effective healthcare, but for those who pay for healthcare, in a time in which need and demand are greater than the resources that are available, optimality is a more appropriate objective. When optimality is achieved, value is at a maximum.

References

(1) Cochrane, A. (1972) Effectiveness and Efficiency: Random Reflections on Health Services. *Nuffield Press (reprinted 2004, RSM)*
(2) Chalmers, I. & Matthews, R. (2006) What are the Implications of Optimism Bias in Clinical Research? *Lancet 367: 449-450*
(3) Kenny, A. (1994) The Wittgenstein Reader. *Blackwell*
(4) Culyer, A. (2005) Healthcare Economics Dictionary. *Cheltenham: Edward Elgar*
(5) Black, N. et al (2006) Health Care Productivity. *BMJ 333: 312-131*
(6) Pearson, S.D. & Rawlins, M.D. (2005) Quality, Innovation and Value for Money: NICE and The British National Health Service. *JAMA 294: 2618-2622*

(7) Henry, D.A. et al (2005) Drug Prices and Value for Money: The Australian Pharmaceutical Benefits Scheme. *JAMA 294: 2630-2632*

(8) Donabedian, A. (2002) An Introduction to Quality Assurance in Health Care. *Oxford Univ. Press*

(9) Donabedian, A. (1980) Explorations in Quality Assessment and Monitoring. (3 vols.) *Health Administration Press*

PART II

THE TOP TEN QUESTIONS ABOUT VALUE

To increase value, those who pay for and manage healthcare, including the hundreds of thousands of clinicians who manage resources as well as looking after individual patients, have to ask ten questions.

(1) **How much money should we spend on healthcare?**

When this is answered, the next question is:

(2) **Is the money allocated for the infrastructure that supports clinical care at a level which will maximise value?**

When this is answered, the next question is:

(3) **Have we distributed the money for clinical care to different parts of the country by a method that recognises both variation in need and maximises value for the whole population?**

When this is answered, the next question is:

(4) **Has money been distributed to different patients groups, e.g. people with cancer or with mental health problems, by decision-making that not only equitable but also maximises value for the whole population?**

When resources have been allocated to a service for a particular group of patients, two further questions have to be asked about the service offered:

(5) **Are all the interventions being offered likely to confer a good balance of benefit and harm, at affordable, for this group of patients?**

(6) **Are the patients most likely to benefit, and least likely to be harmed, from the interventions, clearly defined?**

Finally, having allocated the money to a service manager, four questions have to be asked about the use of resources:

(7) Is effectiveness being maximised?

(8) Are the risks of care being minimised?

(9) Can costs be reduced further without increasing harm or reducing benefit?

(10) Could each patient's experience be improved?

Those who pay for and those who manage healthcare are interested in all these questions. Traditionally the lead is taken by payers for the earlier questions, by those who have direct management responsibility for the later questions with both parties interested in all of them (Figure 4.1).

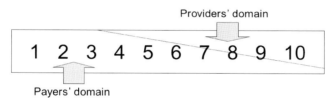

Figure 4.1 *The 20th century relationship between providers and payers*

As pressure increases there is a convergence of interests. On the one hand, those who provide care, and patient groups, are increasingly involved in lobbying for more resources for healthcare. On the other hand, those who pay for healthcare are increasingly involved in assuring and ensuring the quality of care provided through 'pay-for-performance' requirements in their contracts. (Figure 4.2)

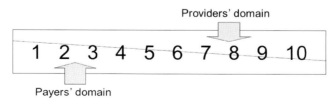

Figure 4.2 *The 21st century relationship between providers and payers*

These questions, and some answers, form the rest of this part of the book.

Question 1

How much money should we spend on healthcare?

There appears to be no limit to the amount of money that can be spent on healthcare. Everyone could have his own personal physician and still want a second opinion. The record is currently held by the United States, which spends more on healthcare, as a proportion of Gross National Product (GNP) than any other large developed country. However, it does this while still leaving 40 million of its population without insurance cover.

One view is that it does not matter how much of the GNP is spent on healthcare because people might as well spend money on health as on holidays or cars, or any other type of conspicuous consumption. It does, however, depend on how the money is raised. If, as in the US, healthcare insurance is part of the employment costs, the increasing cost of insurance affects the costs of American goods and contributes in part to other economic problems.

The amount that is spent on healthcare is a value judgement based on a number of different criteria, for example:

- The proportion of the GNP spent on healthcare in other comparable countries. Comparison with spending in the European Union was an important factor in influencing the Labour government to spend a high proportion of the UK GNP on health.
- Consideration of the opportunity costs of increasing spending on healthcare in comparison with all the other demands on government funds, for example education, defence or law enforcement. Every pound or euro spent on healthcare is a pound or euro that cannot be spent on education, and that is a value decision.
- The relationship between the capacity of the service and public

concern about service shortfall. Concern about waiting times, for example, has driven many countries to increase investment in healthcare, but this type of decision-making, may simply lead to a diversion of resources to the particular service highlighted by the media rather than increasing the amount of GNP allocated to healthcare. The evidence for this approach is weak and one well conducted study found that 'despite more resources physicians in regions of high healthcare intensity did not report greater ease in obtaining needed services or providing high quality care'. (1)

This debate involves macro-economic decisions. In countries like the UK, in which expenditure is either public or private, the decision for those who distribute the public purse is relatively simple, based firstly on a decision about the proportion of the GNP that is to be public expenditure and then the proportion of that expenditure that is to be allocated to healthcare. In many of those countries in which the proportion of the GNP spent on healthcare is greater than 10%, the options are more complex. This is because much of the spend is not from private citizens making a decision to invest in healthcare rather than another holiday, but from insurance schemes subsidised or underwritten by government, which affects the size of public sector spending. In Germany, for example, the insurance companies made a profit of 1.8 billion euros in 2005, but the government had to invest 4.2 billion euros to support the difference between insurance contributions and costs, and a German Minister caused an uproar when he proposed that German citizens spend less on holidays and more on public services.

Where insurance schemes are not supported by public sector spending, they are usually supported by employers, and this affects the price of goods and services produced by the country. In the 1970s, the cost of healthcare insurance became greater than the cost of steel in Chrysler cars. This was not the only problem faced by Chrysler; the quality of their cars was much worse than the quality of Japanese cars, but the combination of cost and quality dealt a heavy blow to Chrysler and to all American car companies from which they have not recovered, and probably never will.

Economists believe that both increases in public sector spending, and increases in the cost of goods and services because of health insurance cost increases, harm the economy of a country and, therefore, in the long-term will impair the health of its population. A Treasury therefore can argue that it is of greater value to the health of a population to control investment in healthcare than to let it run uncontrolled. In most developed countries the Finance Ministry or Treasury, and not the Health Ministry, has decided that not much more than 10% of the GNP should be spent on healthcare.

Reference

(1) Sirovich, B. et al (2006) Regional Variations in Health Care Intensity and Physician Perceptions of Quality of Care. *Ann. Int. Med. 144: 641-649*

Question 2

Is the money allocated for the infrastructure that supports clinical care at a level which will maximise value?

Eyeball to eyeball, clinician and patient: the consultation is at the heart of the patient's experience of healthcare. About 20,000 consultations occur every day in a population of a million.

Many decisions are reached in the consultation by the two protagonists or partners – about 100,000 decisions a day for every million population. Many clinicians also make decisions without directly engaging with the patient, either by providing knowledge from their laboratory or radiology service, or by contributing their expertise in a multi-disciplinary team meeting to which the another clinician has brought the patient's records, but not the patient.

These clinical services are of direct value to patients, provided, of course, that:

- they are doing the right things to
- the right patients and
- doing them right

There are, however, support services which are not clinical: management, education, research and Information Technology (IT). Decisions have to be made about how much money should be allocated for these purposes (Figure Q2.1).

What is the value of management?

Someone has to pay clinicians, buy the equipment they use and carry out a myriad of activities, such as organising the car parking – someone defined a modern hospital as a set of departments united only by

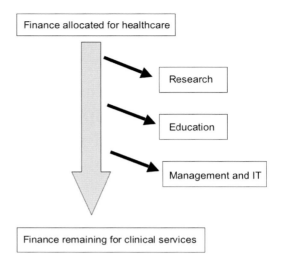

Figure Q2.1 *'Top Slicing' money before the funding of clinical care*

complaints about car parking! Resources have to be invested in management or administration – the term varies from one service to another – but how much of the resources? The answer is as little as is necessary for the effective administration of the service, but there is no evidence-based formula that can be used to answer this question.

There are no randomised trials of health services, with 5% management costs compared to health services with 10% management costs, in part because of the difficulty in defining what is meant by a 'management cost'. It has been argued that healthcare management illustrates Parkinson's Law perfectly – management tasks increase in direct proportion to the amount of management time available to tackle them. (1) The logical conclusion of this principle, a hospital fully staffed with administrators but without a single patient, was compellingly portrayed in the BBC television series *Yes, Minister!* The costs of management increase as the amount of regulation increases, however. If, for example, it is mandated that clinicians must have an externally validated appraisal of their competence each year, a system has to be set up to manage this process, and management costs increase as a consequence, so managers can cannot be blamed for all the increase in the costs of management.

Whatever the proportion of resources spent on management, no-one argues with the fact that some investment is necessary. If all management costs were cut, the service would grind to a halt very quickly. Just how quickly depends on how much stock is available, but in a hospital working on 'lean' principles, with very little stock in the pharmacy, the laboratory, or the linen store, the service would grind to a halt within a week. The same cannot be said for investment in education or research. If such investment were cut, the impact would take longer to manifest.

What is the value of education?

The clinical staff of a health service is the resource that delivers the service to patients. They need buildings and equipment, and management support, but the clinical staff is of central importance in realising the potential benefit that investment in equipment and buildings offers. Where do staff come from?

Health service staff are recruited as a result of investing in an advertisement, but to ensure that there are sufficient trained staff to recruit, a health service has to address that standard business question: 'make or buy?'

The attraction of buying staff is obvious. The service only has to pay the salaries of the staff it employs, and not meet the costs of training. A service should invest a significant sum in the training of replacements, or it can buy the clinical staff produced by another country.

Germany, for example, had a policy of allowing everyone who was qualified to do so to go to university. The predictable result was that it produced an 'Ärzteschwemme' – a flood of doctors – which, when money was plentiful, could of course staff that other German phenomenon, the 'Bettberg' – the bed mountain. As resources became scarcer, medical unemployment and under-employment emerged, and the English NHS was able to meet the need produced by German higher education and health services. This is a simple market issue. There is, however, a moral issue when developed countries buy the professional staff trained by poor countries.

What is the value of research?

The value of investment in research is more complicated. Again, a health service could answer the make or buy question by 'buying' research outputs from other countries, subscribing to journals or the Cochrane Library, or simply by using the free service of PubMed from the National Library of Medicine in the USA, and the increasingly influential free knowledge sources such as the Public Library of Medicine, BioMed Central, and PubMed Central.

The economic benefits

There are, however, a number of reasons why health services would be ill-advised not to invest in the support of research.

- *'The proportion of the most frequently cited articles funded by industry increased over time and was equal to the proportion funded by government or public sources... Academics may be losing control of the research agenda.'* (2)
- *'Conclusions in trials funded by for profit organisations may be more positive due to biased interpretation of trial results.'* (3)
- *'Constraints on the publication rights were described in 40 (91%) of the protocols from 1994/5 and 22 (50%) noted that the [industry] sponsor either owned the data or needed to approve the manuscript or both.'* (4)

If the health service does not invest in research, the evidence base will be increasingly stocked with pharmaceutical research, and if decisions are to be evidence-based there will be increased investment in drugs simply because the evidence base for, to give two examples, walking therapy for arterial disease or psychological therapy for depression, will be much weaker without health service investment.

There is, however, another factor which has to be taken into consideration when deciding how much to invest in research, namely the value that such investment has for the economy of the country as a whole.

If an improvement in the health of the population is regarded as an economic good, as it should be, the return for society from investment in research can be shown to be valuable. A major review of the economic benefits of investing in the US National Institutes of Health (NIH) concluded that 'the public return on investment has been

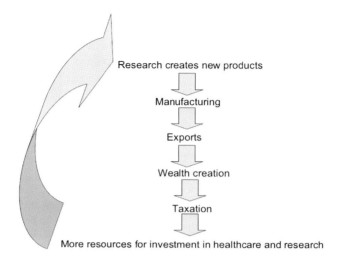

Figure Q2.2 *The benefits of research to the economy*

substantial. Although results have led to increases in healthcare expenditures, health gains were large and valuable.' (5)

If investment in research can be justified, the next question is to ask: how much? The National Health Service Research and Development programme was set up on the recommendation of a House of Lords Committee, with the aim of investing 1.5% of NHS resources in the direct cost of research and the 'support of research'. This support is needed to meet the extra costs in a clinical service in which clinicians are carrying out research. This policy was a necessary consequence of the introduction of a healthcare market because the total costs of care in a hospital with a large research programme were often greater than the costs of care in a hospital with no research.

The debate about the value of research was stimulated in 2006 in the United Kingdom by the decision to review the need for two publicly funded research programmes, one focusing on 'laboratory research', the other focusing on 'practice-orientated research'. Practice-orientated research is a term chosen rather than 'clinical research', which has come to mean laboratory research on the basic mechanisms of disease as opposed to research on how best to prevent or treat disease to-day (6,7). Practice-orientated research can bring rapid benefit to those who manage or pay for healthcare. For example, there has long been uncertainty about the relative merits of venous and arterial catheters in the management of patients with severe trauma. A well designed and executed research project produced an unequivocal answer of immediate use to the healthcare providers and payers:

> *'Pulmonary Artery Catheter (PAC) guided therapy did not improve survival or organ function but was associated with more complications than central venous catheter (CVC) guided therapy. These results, when considered with those of previous studies, suggest that the PAC should not be used routinely for the management of acute lung injury.'* (8)

The value of research to patients

Research results are often of value to patients, but the immediate value of being involved in research is less clear. It is true that it can give the patient the opportunity of a new treatment not routinely available but the new treatments being tested may be ineffective. It is also true that patients in research are looked after very carefully, according to strict protocols. The involvement of children in leukaemia research, for instance, has helped transform that disease from a certain killer to one that is often cured.

For many patients, however, the value of involvement in research is the sense of altruism. The Million Women Collaborative Study in England recruited a million women as they attended for breast cancer screening, who now feel that they are not research subjects, but partners in the war against breast cancer.

How much should be invested in Information Technology to maximise value?

A modern health service cannot run without computers. Some investment is therefore necessary, but how much to maximise value? There is no simple answer.

Costs

The cost of the investment is usually easy to estimate, although the history of IT investment in both industry and the public sector is that, unless the contracts are very carefully drafted, the actual cost is often greater than the planned cost. The National Audit Office review of the NHS Information Technology Programme in England explicitly praises the contracting process, which ensured that contractors stick to the agreed cost.

Administrative benefits

The benefits are easier to describe, but more difficult to measure in financial terms. They can reduce the staffing costs of healthcare administration. of scheduling appointments, but the magnitude of these management savings has never been clearly estimated because:

- computerisation has crept into hospitals piecemeal while, at the same time
- administration has become more complex

Clinical benefits

There is, however, another benefit from IT investment: a clinical benefit for patients. There is good enough evidence that investment in IT can:

- reduce clinical errors
- increase the effectiveness of healthcare by faster uptake of high value interventions
- reduce the harmful effects of healthcare by preventing unknowing prescription of drugs that interact with one another

The evidence is good enough, according to one of the leading innovators and evaluators of healthcare IT, John Halamka. (9) More evidence is needed, particularly about the contribution of clinical decision tools – software that reminds and alerts both clinicians and patients about clinical actions that should or should not be considered, but the evidence that some investment will produce clinical benefit is good enough.

The decision to spend some resources on Information Technology for clinical benefit is not difficult. The difficulty lies in deciding how much, bearing in mind the fact that investment in IT almost certainly is governed (as is so much healthcare investment) by the law of diminishing returns with, at best, a flattening of the curve relating benefit to investment and, probably a point of optimality beyond which the health gain, or net benefit, declines. IT, like all technology, can do harm as well as good. The decision is more complicated than the decision about investment in IT to increase the productivity of administration. The benefits of investment in clinical IT are not 'cash releasing' – that is, they do not allow the number of clinical staff to be reduced. The main justification for investment in clinical IT is that it obviates some of the need for additional senior clinical staff by ensuring that less experienced clinical staff have their decisions guided by clinical pathways, prompts and reminders.

So if asked to come off the fence, what would I advise? I would say that on the evidence available, a knowledge-rich activity like healthcare should invest up to 5% of its resources in information sub-systems. I would emphasise the need to focus on information sub-systems rather than the more commonly used term 'information systems', because investment in information technology is a means to an end, not an end in itself. The end is better clinical care, and information technology can contribute to that end, but there is evidence that if information technology is put in before the clinical systems – the objectives of care, the criteria that allow progress to be measured, the pathways to ensure that objectives will be attained – the investment can do more harm than good.

Putting a computer system into an unstructured mess of consultations and clinical encounters will not, by itself, transform the mess and may increase the confusion. One study showed that mortality increased following the introduction of computerised prescribing (10), which was not attributed to the computer software itself but to the impact of computer screens, and new procedures on team work and clinical judgement.

References

(1) Parkinson, C.N.C. (1958) Parkinson's Law, or the Pursuit of Progress. *Penguin*
(2) Patsopoulos, N. et al (2006) Origin and Funding of the Most Frequently Cited Papers in Medicine. *BMJ* 332: *1061-64*
(3) Als-Nielsen, B. et al (2003) Association of Sources of Funding And Conclusions in Randomised Controlled Trials. *JAMA 290: 921-928*
(4) Gotzsche, P. et al (2006) Constraints on Publication Rights in Industry-initiated Controlled Trials. *JAMA 295: 1645-1646*

(5) Johnston, S.C. et al (2006) Effect of a US National Institutes of Health Programme of Clinical Trials on Public Health. *Lancet 367: 1319-1327*

(6) Horton R (2006) Health Research in the UK; the price of success. *Lancet 368: 93-9*

(7) Rothwell, P.M (2006) Funding for Practice-orientated Research. *Lancet 368: 262-266*

(8) The NHLBI ARDS Clinical Trials Network: PAC versus CVC to Guide the Treatment of Acute Lung Injury (2006) *NEJM 354*: 2213–2224

(9) Halamka, J.D. (2006) Health Information Technology: Shall We Wait for the Evidence? *Ann. Int. Med. 144:775-776*

(10) Han, Y.Y. et al (2005) Unexpected Increased Mortality after Computerized Physician Order Entry System. *Paediatrics 116: 1506-1512*

Question 3

Have we distributed the money for clinical care to different parts of the country by a method that recognises both variation in need and maximises value for the whole population?

Publicly funded healthcare is designed to meet need, and resources are allocated on the basis of need, but the definition of need is not always straightforward, and the quantification of the need of different populations is a complicated issue, which often requires a very simple solution.

In a developed country, the single most important factor is the age of the population served, because most diseases become more common in older age groups. However, allocation on the basis of age alone would be inequitable because there are other factors that determine the health needs of a population, notably poverty. Almost all diseases are more common among poor people. The definition of 'poor' itself is not universally agreed. It can be defined in absolute terms, for example with respect to a certain level of income, or in relative terms, for example with respect to the distribution of income in the population. Furthermore, there is discussion as to whether poverty itself is the only factor or whether deprivation, a sense of alienation and low worth, is a separate variable and needs recognition. In calculating risk for heart disease, for example, the Scottish Executive has identified all the people living in particularly deprived communities as being of high priority, even though all the individuals in those communities may not be very poor.

If the desire is to maximise value by matching resources to need, then resources must be allocated taking into account not only the age distribution of the population but also the level of poverty and deprivation within the community. In the United Kingdom, the simplest approach has been to use the Standardised Mortality Ratio. Obviously, poverty and deprivation cause disability as well as early mortality, but the Standardised Mortality Ratio reflects levels of disability and morbidity within the population and is used as an indicator of health need, either alone or with additional weighting to take into account the poverty of the population.

This is not an exact science. Those representing populations favoured by the formula often feel that the formula does not reflect them sufficiently; those representing populations that are losers on account of the formula may feel, on the other hand and not surprisingly, that the formula employed makes too much allowance for deprivation.

Question 4

Has money been allocated to different patient groups in a way that will maximise value for the whole population?

When clinical care is examined closely, it resembles Brownian motion – a random movement of small particles. From the perspective of a manager or payer, not looking at the care of individual patients but at the care of groups of patients, for example people with mental health problems, lung cancer, or cystic fibrosis, the Brownian motion is not necessarily visible. This is because people who manage and pay for healthcare often look at budget sheets and annual reports and do not sit through clinics, or follow individual patients on their journey through healthcare. It is very important for managers to get a better appreciation of what is happening on the shop floor', 'at the coal face' or 'in the front line' because of the evidence that the major drivers of healthcare cost increases are the increasing volume and intensity of clinical practice – the apparently inexorable trend towards the provision of care, which has:

- more professionals involved
- more tests
- more referrals
- more treatments
- more complex treatment
- more recognition of the need for patient involvement
- more follow-up
- more handovers
- more record-keeping
- more litigation

If we were to arrive in some new, uninhabited world, with no investment at all in healthcare, and were asked to design a health service, life would be relatively, though not completely, straightforward.

Hellish decisions would still have to be made about how much money should be allocated to patients with cancer and how much to people with mental illness.

A few people have had the opportunity to do this when they have been appointed to manage health services in small but very rich states, where a massive increase in investment is planned, but even they often inherit the consequences of years, sometimes decades, of chaotic investment. In most developed countries, the person who comes new to a job managing or paying for healthcare, knows that they are going to inherit a mess. Even the best managed services are messes – using the term 'mess' to mean a management problem for which there is:

- no ideal solution, and for which
- every solution will create further problems

Many payers and providers will be faced with a budget sheet that presents the expenditure as it relates to expenditure to institutions, such as hospital and community services, or relates to expenditure to broad divisions that bear little resemblance to the work of clinicians, for example by presenting information describing expenditure on medicine, surgery, laboratory, and imaging. A person with cancer of the bowel, or almost any other serious problem, will use resources from all four. To answer Question 3 with any validity, it is necessary to organise the budgets on the basis of the health problems that the clinicians are tackling.

The need for Programme Budgeting

Increasingly, the need for organising budgets which focus on programmes of care has been recognized, and the Department of Health in England has defined a set of Programme Budget Categories, based on the International Classification of Disease, to accelerate this trend. The Categories are:

(1) Infectious Diseases, excluding Tuberculosis and Sexually Transmitted Disease
(2) Cancers and Tumours, including those with suspected, or at risk of developing Cancer
(3) Blood Disorders
(4) Endocrine, Nutritional and Metabolic Problems

    (5) Mental Health Problems
    (7) Neurological System Problems
    (8) Vision Problems
    (9) Hearing Problems
    (10) Circulation Problems
    (11) Respiratory Problems, including Tuberculosis and Sleep Apnoea
    (12) Dental Problems, including Preventive Checks and Community Surveys
    (13) Gastro-Intestinal Problems
    (14) Skin Problems
    (15) Musculo-skeletal Problems, excluding Trauma
    (16) Trauma and Injuries, including Burns
    (17) Genito-urinary Problems, excluding Infertility
    (18) Maternity and Reproductive health
    (19) Neonates
    (20) Poisoning
    (21) Healthy Individuals
    (22) Social Care Needs – problems related to life-management difficulty, and problems related to care-provider dependency
    (23) Other

Programme Budgets for individual conditions

Programme budgets can be set at a finer level of granularity, at the level of the specific health problem - for breast cancer, rheumatoid arthritis, or cystic fibrosis, for example. Indeed, Porter and Teisberg, in their analysis (1) of the reasons why competition has failed to deliver high quality healthcare in the United States, argue that it is essential to do this and to encourage competition between 'Integrated Patient Units', delivering care to patients with specific conditions, because competition between hospitals or insurance companies is too broad to have any meaning.

The limitations of Programme Budgeting

It should not be imagined that this approach will clarify all issues: in managing a mess, every solution creates further problems, raising questions such as:

- How do we allocate the cost of care of an old person who has Alzheimer's disease, heart failure and arthritis, and social care needs?
- How should the costs of reaching a diagnosis be allocated?
- How should paediatrics be classified?
- How do we allocate training costs?

In addition, it is essential for the payer to ensure that the programme budget covers all the costs of care. Programme budgeting in a hospital, for example, can lead to behaviour such as the discharge of patients with only enough medication for 48 hours, so as to transfer the costs to another budget. From the payer's perspective, therefore, it is essential to ensure that programme budgets relate to the whole population, covering the costs of treating all the people with rheumatoid arthritis in a particular population. Even this approach does not include costs incurred by patients and carers, unless some of the healthcare resources are given directly to patients or their carers, but a full programme budget should also include these costs.

Annual population value review

Once programme budgets have been defined, the second test of values set out at the head of this chapter can be applied, namely if you want to know someone's values, give them a choice. With a programme-based budget, it is possible to conduct an Annual Population Value Review and, using marginal analysis, test the effect of increasing and decreasing each budget on the value derived from the resources. It is also possible to review the value of each programme.

Is value reduced by hidden inequities?

> *Language constructs reality; it does not reflect it (2)*
> *Equity: the quality of being equal or fair; impartiality; even-handed dealing (3)*

Programme budgeting based on the International Classification of

Disease (ICD) creates what sociologists would call a medical construction of healthcare: nothing wrong with that but it is only one perspective, a health service viewed through a medical lens. Imagine now that the high level classification was not based on the ICD but on gender, or age, ethnic group or socio-economic group. A completely different budget structure would be developed, and different decisions would have to be faced. Instead of asking the question:

- Has money been distributed to different patients groups, e.g. people with cancer or with mental health problems, by decision-making that is equitable and maximises value for the whole population?

Decision-makers would be asking questions such as:

- Has money been distributed to different age groups, e.g. children or adults or elderly people, by decision-making that is equitable and maximises value for the whole population?
- Has money been distributed to meet the different needs of men and women by decision-making that is equitable and maximises value for the whole population?
- Has money been distributed to different ethnic groups, e.g. people from south Asia or from Africa, by decision-making that is equitable and maximises value for the whole population?
- Has money been distributed to different socio-economic groups by decision-making that is equitable and maximises value for the whole population?

There is evidence that if these questions are asked, using these lenses, many health services appear to spend less resources, relative to the needs of the group, on minority ethnic groups, women, older people, poor people, and less well-educated people.

It could be argued that this is the result of issues unrelated to values, for example the literacy of poorly educated people. This, however, ducks the issue. The decision-maker needs to form a judgment about whether healthcare resources should be invested in services specifically for these groups, such as in services for sickle cell disease, or in ancillary services, such as the provision of interpreters which could increase utilisation.

A Programme Budget for children

The allocation of money to children's services poses a particular challenge. The amount of resources allocated to children is difficult to discern because children are treated by every service except geriatrics, yet the only ICD budget heading is 'neonates'. The amount invested in improving the health of children needs to take into account not only the present needs of children but also the values we place on children and their future contribution to society. At a meeting in Oxford's Town Hall, convened to deplore that lack of investment in services for elderly people, the mood of indignation mounted as speaker after speaker called for more resources for the elderly. Then one woman, herself indubitably elderly, stood up and said: 'Let's face it, important though we are, it is children who need the resources.' This was greeted with universal applause, including from those who had called for more resources for older patients.

Tools for Programme Budget analysis

Tools are being developed to appraise options in more detail than simple cost-effectiveness, expressed as a 'cost per QALY'. One approach, called the 'weighted benefit score framework', uses seven criteria, such as 'the effect on quality of life and the preventive impact.' (4) Another approach has been the development of two criteria:

- The Disease Impact Number is the number of people with a disease of whom one will benefit if an intervention were to be offered to all patients.
- The Population Impact Number is the number of people in a particular population who would benefit if the intervention were to be introduced to that population. (5)

These criteria show promise, but have not yet been evaluated in practice.

References

(1) Porter, M. and Teisberg, E. (2006) Redefining Healthcare. *Harvard Bus. School Press*

(2) Whorf, B.L. (1956) Language, Thought and Reality. Selected Writings of Benjamin Lee Whorf. *MIT Press*

(3) Shorter Oxford English Dictionary

(4) Wilson, E.C.F. et al (2006) Developing a Privatisation Framework in an English Primary Care Trust. *Cost Effectiveness and Resource Allocation 4:3*

(5) Heller, R.F. (2005) Evidence for Population Health. *Oxford University Press*

Question 5

Are the interventions being offered all likely to confer a good balance of benefit and harm for this group of patients?

For any group of patients there are many possible interventions that could be offered. These can be classified using the following simple matrix (Figure Q5.1).

	High value	Low value
Provided	A	B
Not provided	C	D

Figure Q5.1 *The imperfect relationship between provision and benefit*

It may be that the service under consideration is providing only the interventions in Box A, and cannot identify any in Boxes B or C: the perfect service. This is not common. Usually it is possible to identify interventions of Type B, C and D. The payer and provider must have a strategy for each of the four situations:

For A - Keep them going, and do them better each year
For B - Start them stopping
For C - Start them starting
For D - Stop them starting

In the 'How To' section of this book, a method is described that can be used to classify all the interventions that are, or could be, provided, to begin a process of:

- increasing the proportion of interventions that are high value
- decreasing the number of interventions that are low value

Appraising a single intervention

When the process of value improvement starts, the debate usually moves quickly, from a consideration of all the interventions that are, or could be, offered to focus on interventions which:

- clinicians and patients want to be introduced
- clinicians and patients want more of
- payers want less of, or want to stop

This leads to the need to have a method for appraising the value of a single intervention and the questions used to appraise new treatments, tests, or services have evolved in the last 30 years.

Is this treatment effective?

This was the question of the 1970s, when the concept of effectiveness had been accepted, and Archie Cochrane's principle that 'all effective treatments must be free' seemed attainable. In the 1980s, concern about the adverse effects of healthcare became much more prominent – not the adverse effects arising from medical errors, but adverse effects inherent in the intervention itself.

Thalidomide was, and still is, the most powerful example of this, because of the obvious side-effects, but there were other dramatically harmful interventions. Many people have minor arrhythmias after a myocardial infarction, and some die when these minor arrhythmias became major. When drugs were developed that controlled some of these arrhythmias they became very popular and were widely used. Unfortunately, the case for introducing these drugs was based on a plausible theory, and some experimental evidence, but the evidence of benefit was not strong, and the evidence of harm was very weak. This was not because there was no harm, but because researchers were focused on the benefits. The 'effects' of the term 'effectiveness' were, at that time, always considered to be good effects, but by the late 1980s those drugs were killing as many as 70,000 people in the United States every year, more than died in the Vietnam War. The saga is described in the book *Deadly Medicine: Why Tens of Thousands of Heart Patients Died in America's Worst Drug Disaster* by Thomas J. Moore. (1) As a consequence, the key question became:

What are the benefits and harms of this intervention?

Evidence about the harms of interventions is less plentiful than evidence of benefit because:

- harms are less common than benefits
- research projects designed to demonstrate the benefits of a new treatment are often not big enough to demonstrate any harm it may cause

Furthermore, during the 1990s, it became clear that the magnitude of the benefits and the harms needed to be expressed in absolute terms. Instead of expressing the results of a trial of a new treatment in relative terms, saying, for example, that the new treatment doubled the cure rate, with only a 10% harm rate, it was clearer both to clinicians and patients if the number of patients receiving a benefit, and the number of patients

	METHOD OF EXPRESSING EFFECTS	
	Relative terms	Absolute terms
Benefits	100% improvement in cure rate	1 in 2,000 patients will be cured instead of 1in 4,000
Harms	50% reduction in the rate of serious adverse effects	5 patients in every 100 die of side effects instead of 10

Figure Q5.2 *Expressing benefits and harms in absolute and relative terms*

being harmed were clearly described in absolute terms, or numbers, and not in percentages (Figure Q5.2)..

There is evidence that if a patient (2), doctor (3), or payer (4), is given information in relative percentage terms, they are keener to use the new treatment than if the same data is presented in absolute terms. This phenomenon, called 'framing', is, of course, well recognised by those who wish to promote new tests and treatments. Also in the 1990s cost became a massive issue for all services, so the key questions became:

Does this treatment do more good than harm at reasonable cost?

This raises the question of judging the reasonableness of cost, and cost benefit analysis was introduced. Economic evaluation was widely introduced, using the cost per quality adjusted life year as criterion, and NICE (The National Institute of Clinical Excellence in England) expressed the results of economic studies in the following way (Figure Q5.3.)

Cost per QALY	Recommendation
Less than $30,000	Cost effective
$30,600 to $45,900	"Likely to be recommended as cost effective"
Over $45,900	"Unlikely to be recommended as cost effective"

Figure Q5.3 *NICE criteria*

One of the reasons for this book is the recognition that many societies now have more requests for funding cost effective interventions that have passed the test of reasonableness, than they can afford to fund, so the question now becomes:

Does this treatment do more good than harm at affordable cost?

This implies that the payer, or the person managing the service, has a piggy-bank full of money just waiting for such an occasion. The manager may bid to the payer for funding in the expectation that the budget will be increased if the case is good, but an increase in budget for one group of patients will, except in times or steady growth, lead the payer, or the manager of a large service faced with a bid from one department, to ask:

Should we move money from another programme budget to meet the costs of this innovation?

The first response of the payer or manager should, however, be the question:

Is this new treatment, or test, of greater value than some other intervention being offered to this group of patients?

Clinicians are already quite good at ditching low value interventions in order to accommodate higher value interventions, but the process needs to become faster and more focused to get better value healthcare.

References

(1) Moore, T.J. (1995) Deadly Medicine: Why Tens of Thousands of Heart Patients Died in America's Worst Drug Disaster. *Simon & Schuster.*
(2) Hux, J.E. and Naylor, C.D. (1995) Does the Format of Efficacy Data Determine Patients' Acceptance of Treatment? *Medical Decision Making 15: 152-157.*
(3) Malenka, D.J. et al (1993) The Framing Effects of Absolute and Relative Risk. *J. Gen. Int. Med 8: 543-548*
(4) Fahey, T. et al (1995) Evidence-based Purchasing. *BMJ* 311: *1056-1060*
(5) Pearson, S.D. and Rawlins, M.D. (2005) Quality, Innovation and Value for Money: NICE and the British National Health Service. *JAMA 294: 2618-2622*

Question 6

Are the patients most likely to benefit, and least likely to be harmed from the interventions, clearly defined?

The simplest answer is that the patients most likely to benefit are similar are those whose clinical condition is exactly the same as that of the patients in the research which produced the evidence that led to the decision to introduce the treatment. For example, the Abtacept trial found that the drug was effective in patients with rheumatoid arthritis who had an 'inadequate response to Methotrexate'. Thus, only patients with an inadequate response to Methotrexate should be given Abtacept. (1)

Once the intervention becomes widely used, however, adherence to these criteria is not always strictly observed and the criteria often drift, which may be driven by clinicians, patients, or industry, or all three.

Technology driven drift

'Don't let those bloody physicians get their hands on the kidney!' This was the only advice I received from the head of the Department of Surgery when I started work as a junior doctor. To my surprise, I had discovered that the Department of Surgery was responsible for acute dialysis for their region, and that I was not only one of the team that would run it, but also that, when the only other member of the team, a Senior Registrar of great experience and competence, went off to operate in another city, I was the team!

And so we dialysed! Almost every night, when the day job was finished, we wheeled out the kidney, a silver cylinder about the size of a dustbin, filled it with water from the tap, turned on the heating element, poured in bags of sodium chloride, glucose, and other mixers in smaller amounts, and stirred the mixture with what is known in Scotland as a 'spurtle' – a wooden stick with a thistle carved at the top for stirring porridge – until the salts dissolved, and the solution was warm enough. At this point we connected the patient to the machine, wrote up the night's plan, and went to bed, perchance to sleep! It was a very successful service.'

When resources are as limited as they were when there was one artificial kidney for a million people, the decision to dialyse was not difficult. In a small number of patients, acute renal failure is temporary, and if they are supported for a period of time, kidney function is regained and patients no longer need dialysis. The introduction of a single artificial kidney to a population that does not have one therefore adds great value. Young people, who would probably have died before the arrival of the kidney dialysis machine, do not die. I say probably because some people recover kidney function spontaneously and some of our 'successes' were not attributable to our activity as doctors, although the patients always gave us the credit.

Imagine now that the number of artificial kidneys were increased from one to ten. The indications for dialysis would change: in addition to dialysing only young fit people with a high chance of recovery, other older, less fit patients with more severe kidney disease or with other health problems would be accepted for dialysis. There would be some increase in value, but it would not be tenfold. Imagine now that the number of kidneys for transplant were increased from 10 to 50. The same phenomenon would be observed (Figure Q6.1).

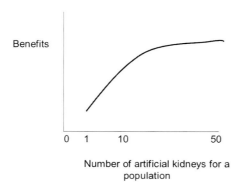

Figure Q6.1 *The Law of Diminishing Returns*

Clinician driven drift

The strict criteria appear to be clear cut, but what often occurs is that, although an intervention is introduced with a very strict definition of which patients should be treated, clinicians gradually drift away from these criteria and extend the indications for intervention to advocate. Patients whose response to Methotrexate was not as good as expected, for example, should be treated with Abtacept, or that Abtacept be used as well as Methotrexate, with the result that patients are treated who do not match the original criteria.

Clinicians hate disease. They want to see patients improve if it is biologically plausible.

Patient driven drift

> *'I operated on the cataract of the retired professor of Pathology. He was delighted. His golf handicap dropped by two. In the following two months, five other members of his golf club were referred for cataract surgery.'*
>
> *(Consultant Opthalmologist)*

When cataract surgery was first introduced, the results were amazing. People with very little vision, some even registered blind, were operated on. As the capacity for cataract surgery increased, the criteria for operation changed. People with less severe degrees of visual loss had their cataracts removed. The cataract operation entered common knowledge, and among older people, demand grew and the early strict criteria started to drift. Patient demands increase as interventions become less unpleasant or less risky.

Drift due to better acceptability

As diagnostic tests become less uncomfortable, they are used on more patients. CT scanning, for example, is less uncomfortable and less risky than the insertion of catheters to arteries for conventional x-ray, so it is judged appropriate to investigate people whose symptoms are less severe.

Drift due to risk reduction

As the adverse effects of treatments diminish, for example as laparascopic ('keyhole') surgery replaces open surgery for removal of the gall bladder, clinicians and patients may accept an operation which they would not previously have done. As the risk of surgery decreases, more people are judged to be 'fit for surgery', so the number of operations with a lower relative risk increases, but the absolute number of deaths remains constant (Figure Q6.2).

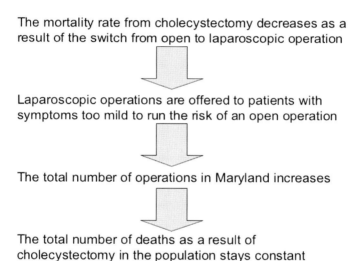

The mortality rate from cholecystectomy decreases as a result of the switch from open to laparoscopic operation

Laparoscopic operations are offered to patients with symptoms too mild to run the risk of an open operation

The total number of operations in Maryland increases

The total number of deaths as a result of cholecystectomy in the population stays constant

Figure Q6. 2 *The impact of changing the threshold for an operation*

As care becomes better organised and of better quality, often as a result of the development of specialist centres, the risks associated with treatment fall, and patients who were previously considered to be too unwell for treatment are reclassified as eligible for treatment.

Industry driven drift

Individual companies try to increase market share, but an industry as a whole may lobby for a particular condition or treatment to be given priority. Direct advertising of a drug or product is one obvious method. In countries in which 'direct to consumer' advertising of drugs is not allowed, healthcare industries – either alone or in concert – have started to fund patient groups, campaigning for more resources for a particular health need, such as female incontinence or osteoporosis. In addition, celebrities who have personal experience of a disease, either as patients or carers, may be recruited to act as figureheads, thus attracting press interest.

From under-use to over-use

Healthcare interventions can be classified as being either necessary or discretionary. Necessary interventions are those over which there is no debate, for example:

- treatment of acute appendicitis, or
- stabilisation of a fractured femur

The decision about whether or not to intervene is straight-forward, provided that the necessary resources are available.

Discretionary interventions are those in which the decision whether or not to intervene rests with the doctor and the patient. Examples of this are:

- psychotherapy
- repair of damaged ligaments in people who are not engaged in professional sport
- admission to hospital of patients with heart failure

When a new technology or service of proven benefit is introduced, it is usually under-used. This can be defined as a failure to provide the service or technology to those patients who have the same characteristics as the patients in the trial from which the evidence emerged that led to the decision to introduce the service. The increased investment of resources to provide the service to all who could benefit will be of value, (although how much value depends, of course, on the other needs that could be met with those resources). There will come a point in time when all the patients who have the same characteristics as the patients in the trial are receiving the service. This can be described as the optimum level of use of the technology. When it is judged that there is over-use of technology, the adjective 'inappropriate' is often used, but inappropriateness is a value judgement.

For payers and providers of care, variations in the rate of interventions are an indicator of over- and under-use, and the *Annual Report* of England's Chief Medical Officer for 2005 contained a whole chapter on the need to tackle variation, entitled 'Waste Not, Want Not'. (2)

Reducing inappropriate clinical practice

Over-use at a population level results from what is called inappropriate clinical practice, but it is very difficult for clinicians to know that they are being inappropriate when face to face with a patient.

The appropriateness of care provided to an individual patient or group of patients can be determined in several different ways:

- by asking an independent clinician or group of clinicians and patients to pass judgement in the intervention given
- by comparing the intervention given to a patient with clinical guidelines indicating which patients are most likely to benefit, or are least likely to be harmed, by that intervention

As the distinction between appropriateness and inappropriateness is a matter of judgement, there is a spectrum of potential categories. In many studies of appropriateness, three categories are identified:

- clearly appropriate
- clearly inappropriate
- a class in between where clinicians, experts and patients disagree, depending upon their values

The concept of appropriateness is particularly useful when making decisions about what Naylor has called the 'grey zones of clinical practice', namely aspects of care for which the evidence is scarce, or the evidence available is not relevant to the patient or the service under consideration. (3)

References

(1) Kremer, J.L. et al (2006) Effects of Abtacept in Patients with Methotrexate-resistant Active Rheumatoid Arthritis. *Ann. Int. Med. 144: 865-876*

(2) Donaldson, Sir Liam (2006) On the State of The Public Health: Annual Report of the Chief Medical Officer 2005. *Department of Health*

(3) Naylor, C.D. (1995) The Grey Zones of Clinical Practice. *Lancet 345: 840-842*

Question 7

Is effectiveness being maximised?

People who manage healthcare resources are not usually involved in answering the first three of the value questions:

- How much money should be spent on direct healthcare?
- How much money should be on research and education?
- How should money be allocated to different populations?

Healthcare managers are involved in decisions to allocate resources to different groups of patients because the force of their argument, often reflecting the power of the clinicians in that specialty, influences resource allocation. Managers are also closely involved with payers in deciding what resources and interventions should be provided for a particular group of patients, and which types of patients are most likely to benefit from those interventions – the fourth, fifth and sixth value questions. The final four questions are primarily the responsibility of people who manage healthcare, although the introduction of 'pay for performance' has brought policy makers and payers much more into the quality debate.

Those who manage healthcare now have their own set of questions to answer, if they are to live up to the 20th century proverb that management consists of only two tasks: 'Doing the right things, and doing them right.' The modern manager must be able to answer, both to their payer, and to the patients and populations they serve, questions 7, 8, 9, and 10 in Chapter 4:

- Is the effectiveness of care being maximised?
- Are the risks of care being minimised?
- Can costs be reduced further without increasing harm or reducing benefit?
- Could each patient's experience be improved?

The 21st century has added a twist to the old proverb because managers are not only expected to do things right, they are expected to do things better and better each year and answer the supplementary questions:

- Are we doing better than last year?
- How do we plan to do even better next year?

Choose the right things to do

The first step in maximising effectiveness is to introduce only those interventions for which there is strong evidence that they will do more good than harm. However, the effectiveness of a health service – 'the degree to which attainable improvements in health are, in fact, attained' (1) – is achieved not only by deciding to provide interventions for which there is strong research evidence of benefit, (that is answering question 5 correctly), but also by ensuring that the benefit demonstrated in the research project which produced the evidence leading to the decision to introduce the service, is actually reproduced in practice.

The second step in maximising effectiveness is, therefore, to introduce only new interventions that are within the capacity of the service to deliver.

Ensure the right things can be well done in an ordinary service setting

The magnitude of the benefit demonstrated in the research setting is sometimes called the efficacy of an intervention, but research is usually done by people who:

- are highly committed
- have special interest and expertise
- work to highly defined protocols
- have their performance continually measured
- have resources earmarked for the work

In the busy service setting, however, these advantages do not exist, and the quality of care may be lower, which means that the magnitude of benefit is lower (Figure Q7.1).

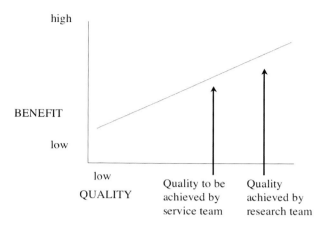

Figure Q7.1 *The difference between the quality of service and research settings*

It is, therefore, not enough to answer question 5 (are the interventions being offered all likely to confer a good balance of benefit and harm?). Particularly when being pressed by an enthusiastic clinician, keen to introduce a new operation or service about which he has either read, or heard at a conference, it is also essential to ask:

- Does this service have, or could it develop, the skills and resources to achieve a level of quality high enough to produce sufficient benefit to justify the investment of resources?

If it is not possible to achieve this level of quality, it does not make sense to introduce the service. Some interventions are easier to introduce, with the confidence that the amount of benefit shown in research can be reproduced. The introduction of a new Statin, which would lower cholesterol more effectively, is easy. The introduction of a new surgical operation, requiring high levels of skill and long experience, or a screening programme, requiring high levels of programme management, is much more challenging. (2)

To manage the introduction of new services in this way requires:

- a system for controlling the introduction of new technology
- a system for managing the introduction of new services

When services are in place, it is then necessary to ensure that each improves year after year after year, and this is done by:

- creating a system for each service
- comparing the performance of each service against explicit standards
- helping each service improve their performance
- resetting the standards regularly

This is the process of continuous quality improvement.

Creating systems

A system is a set of activities with a common set of objectives. Each service must have both a broad aim and a set of objectives.

The aim of the NHS Abdominal Aortic Aneurysm Programme, for example, was defined as being to reduce the mortality from rupture of the aorta. Its specific objectives were defined as follows:

- To offer all men screening in the year following their 65th birthday.
- To men offered screening, to provide information in a language and at a level that suits their needs.
- To ensure that men accepting or refusing screening had an accurate understanding of the benefits and risks involved.
- To measure the abdominal aortic diameter accurately in two dimensions, using designated ultrasound machines.
- To provide continuing surveillance for men whose aortic diameter is over 30mm but less than 55mm.
- To refer all men with an aortic diameter in excess of 55mm to a centre that is part of a nationally recognised network.
- To minimise anxiety.
- To minimise harm.
- To provide support for staff involved in the programme.
- To be accountable to the population served.
- To promote and support research.

For each objective, one or more criteria must be chosen in order to allow progress, or the lack of it, to be measured. This is a system, sometimes called a programme.

Comparing the service with other services

In requiring managers to do better year after year, it necessary to be clear about the yardstick. It is obviously meritorious for a service to do better than it did the previous year, but that is not sufficiently rigorous, because a service could improve from being 'very dangerous' to being 'dangerous' and still meet this criterion. It is essential for a service to compare itself with other services.

Fortunately, the term 'average' has come to have a meaning that implies value, as well as its original statistical meaning, and for a service to boast that it was 'above average' would impress few patients or payers. Furthermore, the average level of performance could be unacceptably poor, and 'above average' could also be unacceptable. For this reason, performance has to be compared with standards.

Comparing the system with standards

> *'The quality of a health service is the degree to which it conforms to pre-set standards of goodness.'*
> *Avedis Donabedian*

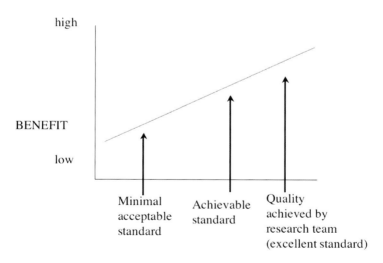

Figure Q7.2 *Different levels of quality*

Standards are subjective. They are value statements. What the manager regards as a good quality service may be regarded as one of very poor quality by the patient, or vice versa. A patient may regard the service as one of very high quality, whereas the payer may regard it as of unacceptably low quality. One reason for this is that each may be considering different aspects of the service, each of which has a quality, and different organisations describe the aspects of the service in different ways, although there are similarities.

The best way to set standards is to decide, on the basis of levels of performance described in the research reports and, if available, data from other services, what would be:

- a minimum acceptable standard, below which no service should be allowed to operate
- an achievable standard to which all services can aspire, and which some will easily surpass (Figure Q7.3)

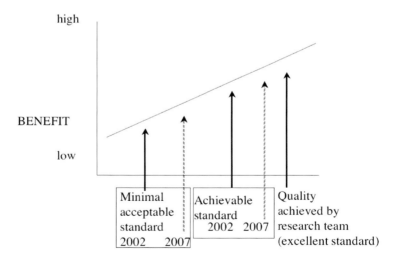

Figure Q7.3 *The re-setting of standards, showing how the achievable standard of the service approaches the level of excellence achieved by the original research team*

Regular resetting of standards for continuous improvement

*'If standards are not being changed annually, it is proof they
are not being used.'*

Kauro Ishikawa:
Total Quality Control – The Japanese Way

Part of quality assurance is the regular resetting of standards, to
prevent boredom and complacency, even though providers may
complain about the constant shifting of the goalposts.

The use of the methods of continuous quality improvement leads
to steady improvement in performance. All services have to be involved
in a process of continuous quality improvement, until the payer decides
that the added value of further improvement of a service is less valuable
than the investment of resources in another service.

References

(1) Donabedian, A. (2002) An Introduction to Quality Assurance in Healthcare. *Oxford University Press.*

(2) Meakins, J. and Gray, J.A.M. (2005) Evidence-Based Surgery. *Surgical Clinics of North America.*

Question 8

Are clinical risks being minimised?

'Punters, we just call them punters, because – let's face it –
they are taking a chance every time they use the health
service!'

A punter is someone who takes a gamble. In a debate at a serious, if
slightly pompous meeting in Belfast about what the people who use
health services should be called – should it be patients or consumers?
– this was the sensible suggestion of one of the doctors. It was his
contribution to the debate about what the people who use health services
should be called – should it be patients or consumers? A punter, one
who takes a gamble, is a serious and respectful term.

All healthcare can cause harm. Everyone who uses health services
runs the risk of harm, but this harm affects not only the patient but also
clinicians, managers, and payers. Harm reduces value.

There are two types of harm:

- harm caused by doing the right thing badly
- harm caused by doing the wrong thing: errors

The harm that results from poor quality healthcare, and the harm
that results from errors are, however, inter-related, because errors are
less likely to occur in high quality services. (1)

Harm caused by doing the right thing badly

Cutting off the wrong leg is an error; cutting off the correct leg, but
doing it so badly that the patient needs a second operation, is harm from
poor quality care.

Because both benefit and this type of harm are functions of the
quality of care provided, the higher the quality of care the better the

69

balance between benefit and harm. There is also a level of quality at which the harms are greater than the benefits.

At this point – the minimal acceptable level of quality – the service should be stopped.

Harm caused by doing the wrong things: errors

An operation on the wrong side of the body, or the prescription of a drug to which the patient is known to be allergic, are errors. Mistakes happen, but the number of mistakes can be minimised.

Preventing errors by continuous quality improvement

Services become high quality for a number of reasons, many of which are factors which have been shown to reduce the incidence of errors, notably:

- good leadership, and
- development of systems

To maximise the probability of benefit and minimise the probability of harm and errors, the professionals need 'Standard Operating Procedures', defined in Wikipedia on 3 August 2006 as 'a procedure, or set of procedures, to perform a given operation or evolution in reaction to a specific event.'

In his annual report for 2005, The Chief Medical Officer (CMO) for England, Professor Sir Liam Donaldson, emphasised the need for Standard Operating Procedures (SOPs). (2) He said that SOPs had a major contribution to make to patient safety, but he recognised that SOPs – 'doing everything exactly the same way all the time' was 'counter-cultural in healthcare.' By that, he meant counter to the culture of clinical autonomy. The challenge was illustrated by the story of an encounter with a surgeon, who told Sir Liam: 'If you introduce that approach, it will be like working in a factory, not being a doctor.' The CMO replied robustly that there is new evidence from many specialties that Standard Operating Procedures are 'compatible with high quality clinical practice by highly trained, highly skilled professionals who continue to exercise judgement in vast areas of their practice.'

Preventing errors by targeted programmes

To improve the quality of safety, it is necessary to have a style of general management designed to improve, which will in turn increase effectiveness and reduce harm, for example:

- promotion of safety culture
- use of systems, including SOPs
- clear lines of accountability for risk management & safety
- data collection about risk factors, errors and near misses

It is also necessary to have risk management targeting those activities or environments where errors are most common and serious, for example:

- high risk activities
  - prescribing
  - handover of care from one clinician to another
  - patient identification

- high risk areas
  - intensive Care
  - operating Theatres
  - emergency Departments

In addition, when new hazards about adverse events and near misses are identified through research, or through the collection and analysis of information, the organisation needs to respond quickly and sensitively, meeting the concerns of the patient who has been harmed, and reducing the risk that other patients could be harmed in the same way. This is what many patients want when harm occurs.

References

(1) Institute of Medicine (2000) To Err is Human: Building a Safer Health System. *National Academies Press*
(2) Donaldson, L. (2006) On the State of the Public Health: Annual Report of the Chief Medical Officer 2005. *Department of Health*

Question 9

Can costs be cut further without increasing harm or reducing effectiveness?

After a business dinner, good food, plentiful drink and bonhomie, it is usually time for a welcome night's sleep. It was a different ending to the story, however, when, at a business dinner, Taiichi Ohno, the recently retired creator of the Toyota production system, finally agreed to advise an American company on how to reduce waste. Any thought of rest was postponed! To the host's 'See you in the morning!' Ohno replied that, if they were serious, they should make an immediate start: call in staff, reorganize the production line, ignore the possible protests of unions. This they did! Ohno moved from the dinner table to the shop floor – jackets off, sleeves up, machinery moved, waste slashed, and productivity increased. (1)

The Japanese term 'kaizen', meaning continual gradual improvement, is now part of the management vocabulary. The term 'muda', meaning waste, is less well-known. Ohno hated waste, defined as 'any human activity which consumes resources but produces no value.' Taiichi Ohno, who has been called the most ferocious hater of waste in history, described seven categories of waste in industrial systems and listed them as:

- Over-production
- Waiting time
- Transportation
- Wasteful processing
- Too much stock
- Too much movement in the factory floor
- Defective products

Ohno's work, and his concept of 'lean thinking' which flowed from it, is of central importance to those who pay for, or manage, health services, but there are some important differences about healthcare, in particular the need to distinguish between productivity and efficiency. (3)

Good outcomes and high productivity are not mutually exclusive

The outcome of healthcare can only be measured by examining and listening to patients. Examples of good outcomes are:

- survival
- cure
- reduced disability

Efficiency relates the outcomes of to what economists call the Inputs, which can be money, staff, beds or other resources. Efficiency is calculated by the formula:

$$\text{Efficiency} = \frac{\text{Outcomes}}{\text{Inputs}}$$

Productivity is simpler to measure. It relates the process of care, the Outputs in the economists' terms, to the Inputs. Productivity is calculated by the formula:

$$\text{Productivity} = \frac{\text{Outputs}}{\text{Inputs}}$$

The efficiency of a cataract service is demonstrated by the number of people able to drive again after cataract removal. The productivity is the number of cataract operations per bed.

The outcomes of care are determined by the interventions used and the quality of the service provided and resources are wasted if a service is not using the:

- right interventions to treat the

- right patients in the
- right way.

The seven steps to improve productivity

Those who pay for and manage the service that is doing the right things, to the right patients, can address the seven causes of low productivity in health services:

(1) Under-use of buildings and equipment
(2) Too much stock
(3) Too much cost for non-essential non-clinical staff
(4) Too much wasted time, for clinicians *and* patients
(5) Care in hospital instead of at home
(6) Staff too skilled, and scarce for the task in hand
(7) Equipment and tools of unnecessary expense

A question and answer for each cause is offered below.

(1) *Can we make more use of buildings and equipment?*

'Sweat the assets' is an industrial proverb, meaning use buildings and plant to the maximum.

- Many Health Centres in the United Kingdom are shut for 115.5 hours in the week.
- Many MRI machines are not used for more than one third of the time.

Staff, of course, have rights, but if a smaller proportion of staff worked from 8.00 a.m. to 6.00 p.m. five days a week, much greater use could be made of fixed assets.

(2) *Can we carry less stock?*

'*In 2005, 574 different head and socket combinations were used in (hip replacement) operations in England and Wales.*

> *It seems implausible that meaningful data can be gathered,
> or that money can be saved through bulk purchase, when
> such a number of products and supplies is used in this way.'*
> *(Annual Report of the Chief Medical*
> *Officer for England, 2005)*

Just-in-time delivery of the equipment needed was one of the great achievements of the Toyota Productions Systems. Most health services buy:

- too much equipment of
- too many types, and
- store it for too long

Such waste can be prevented, and cured, by better procurement.

(3) *How can we reduce the cost of essential non-clinical staff?*

Clinical staff see patients, or samples of patients. They need technical staff, catering, supplies, and laundry, and they need administration and management staff. Different approaches have been taken to reduce costs, for example:

- Outsourcing of non-clinical services to reduce staff costs, because many private contractors pay lower wages or provide less benefits than public service employers, which can be viewed as a moral, as well as a productivity issue.
- Reducing the number of tasks that administrative staff have to do, for example by reducing demands for data
- Reducing the number of management staff
- Reorganisation

Of these methods, the last appears the least effective, and may increase costs in both the short- and the long-term.

(4) *Can the waste of clinician and patient time be reduced?*

Time is the scarcest resource for clinicians. For most clinicians, the highest value work time is that spent on clinical work, followed by research, and then education.

Some of the 'other activities' may have high value, for example if a physician is reimbursed for half a day to reward the time spent in managing resources, but much is, in the everyday phrase, a waste of time, examples of which are:

- meetings without purpose or conclusion
- looking for lost notes or data
- getting a new identity card or parking space

All clinicians have their own lists of what they consider to be a waste of time, but their valuations may not be shared. Attendance at a management meeting may be classified as a waste of time by the clinician, but regarded as high value by a manager. It would require independent evaluation to determine whether the clinician was correct, and the meeting was unfocused and unproductive, or whether the manager's perspective, that the clinician came to a good meeting with the wrong attitude, was correct.

Education and research can also be unproductive and of low value. Education is of low value if:

- it is not determined by the formally ascertained learning needs of the clinician, as opposed to their wants. There is evidence that if clinicians are interested in a topic and want to learn, they will seek out the learning they need. Expenditure on formal training should be reserved for topics for which the clinician is not delivering good quality care.
- it is not delivered using methods which have evidence of effectiveness – large lectures are usually of low value

Research is of low value if:

- the answer is already known
- the design is inappropriate or inadequate
- the conduct of the research is sloppy
- the reporting is biased

Clinical practice is of high value, but within the course of clinical work the time of clinicians and patients is often wasted, if:

- the patient's notes are missing
- key data, such as laboratory results, are not available

- there is unnecessary waiting time, such as between operations in a theatre

(5) *Is care being delivered in the most appropriate place?*

Many patients are treated in facilities which have levels of staffing and equipment which they do not need.

- 'Bed blockers' are patients, usually elderly, who have recovered from the acute phase of their disease but cannot be discharged because they are now too disabled to return home, but unable to be placed in a nursing home. This is a matter of concern both for those who manage or pay for care, and for the patients themselves, who are at high risk of hospital-acquired infection, institutionalisation, and malnutrition.
- Patients who attend a clinic with a problem that might have been resolved if their primary care clinician could have phoned, e-mailed, or had other means of accessing the expertise of the specialist.

The 'Five Whys?' of Taiichi Ohno (see page 94) are worth asking frequently in healthcare.

(6) *Could this care be provided by less highly trained staff?*

Highly trained staff are scarce, and it is a waste of their time to carry out tasks which could be managed equally well by staff who have not had the training to carry out all the tasks of the highly skilled person, but who have been trained specifically to carry out a finite range of tasks. Sometimes such staff carry out repetitive tasks with greater attention to detail, and with better results than the most highly trained staff to whom such tasks are, at best, boring or, at worst, a waste of time.

(7) *Can we procure good equipment and drugs more cheaply?*

When asked what passed through his mind the minute before take-off, the astronaut replied: 'I could not stop thinking that I am sitting on top of the cheapest tender!'

Some people prefer the term 'low cost' to 'cheap', and 'lower cost' to 'cheaper', but who cares about the niceties of language, the key question is why pay more than is necessary? Costs can be reduced by:

- skilful procurement
- bulk purchase
- the use of generic rather than branded drugs
- sometimes 'making' rather than 'buying'

These activities are ethically important because they reduce waste, increase productivity, and release resources for clinical care.

Beyond large scale production

This is the subtitle of Taiichi Ohno's short (143 pages) classic on *The Toyota Production System*, emphasising that one of the cleverest things that Kiichiro Toyoda, the President, and Ohno did was not to overtake the Ford Motor Company with even larger scale production but by small scale production, with less stock and less waste and more flexibility. (2) This not only made good sense but allowed the company to evolve by customer pull, rather than by factory push. Toyota makes personalised cars when an order is placed, so combining industrial production methods and personalisation can lead to success in the manufacturing industry, and also in healthcare. Becoming more productive does not mean becoming less personal.

References

(1) Liker, J. (2004) The Toyota Way. *McGraw Hill*
(2) Ohno, T. (1995) The Toyota Production System. *Productivity Press*
(3) Womack, J.P. and Jones, D.T. (1996) Lean Thinking. *Simon & Schuster*

Question 10

Could each patient's experience be improved?

To the clinician, the management of disease becomes, to some extent, routine. To the patient, the experience is unique and dramatic, with both clinically significant and insignificant incidents etched on memory. Three types of experience have been described, each distinct but all inter-related (Figure Q10.1).

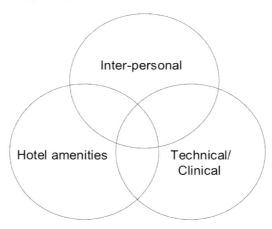

Figure Q10.1 *The factors which determine the patient's experience*

The hotel experience

Hotel factors, such as food and car parking, can be judged by every patient, who will use as their yardstick a hotel they know, or a business they have visited. However, it is difficult for hospitals that accept all comers, planned admissions, and emergencies, to give the appearance of calm prosperity exuded by hotels. Hospitals that specialise only in planned or elective care can maintain or acquire the atmosphere of a good hotel, with flowers, and carpets on the floor, but in a busy general hospital it is more difficult to disguise what it is – a place where life and death, conflict and drama, violence and sorrow, vomit and blood, are on stage day and night.

As a result of the increasing incidence of hospital-acquired infections, one hotel factor of great importance is cleanliness. Using the patient's experience to monitor cleanliness, and patient pressure to improve overt cleanliness, contributes to the prevention of hospital-acquired infections.

With the exception of cleanliness, hotel factors are not a major determinant of patients' rating of the value of their care. If amenities such as car parking are unsatisfactory, they will annoy and irritate, but if they are excellent they will not necessarily lead to delight - people can put up with unappetising food, but rudeness and insensitivity are much more difficult to reconcile.

The inter-personal experience

Politeness is important but can cover a multitude of sins. The relationship between the respect shown to patients and the technical quality of care has not been clearly described but:

- it would not be unreasonable to expect a positive correlation between the technical quality of a service and the respect shown to patients. Feelings of respect are of no value unless they are demonstrated in practice;
- 'feeling respected as an individual' is an outcome that patients value highly and is of value in its own right, independent of the technical outcome of care. Indeed for people with untreatable or incurable problems, it is the only outcome.

It is essential, therefore, to measure the patient's experience of the interpersonal aspects of care as well as measuring their hotel experience. Increasingly there is also interest in measuring the outcome of care from the patient's perspective.

The technical experience

Patients judge the technical quality of their care by the outcome, but high quality care does not necessarily guarantee good outcome. Some patients have a good outcome from poor quality care, and some patients have a bad outcome from good quality care

Studies have shown that, not surprisingly, patients found it difficult to judge the technical quality of care. (1, 2) It is possible for patients to assess the quality of care, provided they have the opportunity to read the annual report of the service, and compare the data with reports of similar services, particularly if the report includes not only measures of activity but also outcomes of value to patients. (3) However, individual patients rarely have access to this type of data at present and usually base their assessment on hotel and interpersonal aspects of their care. This will change, however, as outcomes of value to patients will be used by both those who pay for, and those who manage, care as routine measures of performance.

Measuring outcomes of value to patients

The outcomes of interest to clinicians and researchers have not always been identical to the outcomes of interest to patients.

The involvement of patients in the design of research improves the quality and relevance of the research, by ensuring that outcomes of interest to patients are included in the study. Furthermore, it is sometimes possible to adopt, or adapt, the outcome measure employed in the research for use in routine clinical practice and healthcare management. It is also possible to give patients their care pathway, for example for the management of a chronic condition, not only so that they can be an even more effective co-ordinator of their care, as only the patient is constant in modern healthcare, but also to clarify their responsibilities.

References

(1) Chang, J.T. et al (2006) Patients' Global Ratings of their Healthcare are not Associated with the Technical Quality of their Care. *Ann. Int. Med. 144 665-672*

(2) Rao, M. et al (2006) Patients' Own Assessment of Quality of Primary Care

Compared with Objective Records Based on Measures of Technical Quality of Care. *BMJ 333: 19-22*

(3) Porter, M. and Teisberg, E. (2005) Redefining Healthcare. *Harvard Bus. School Press*

PART III

THE BETTER VALUE
HEALTHCARE TOOLKIT

No matter how senior you may be in the Royal Engineers, it is necessary always to carry with you a small notebook called *The Tactical Aide-Mémoire*. It contains all you must remember, the simple things that are so easy to forget when one gets more senior, partly because of age, and partly because of familiarity with the task. *The Tactical Aide-Mémoire* helps ensure that the officer does not build a bridge that would not carry a tank or, even worse, not reach the other side of a ravine.

Based on this principle, we have developed a set of *Aides-Mémoire* for the manager or payer who is called upon to do the healthcare equivalent of throwing a bridge across a ravine. The pages can be reduced on a photocopier to Filofax size or downloaded from our website, www.bettervaluehealthcare.org/book/howtodoit.

HOW TO RESPOND TO A BID FOR A NEW TREATMENT OR SERVICE

WHY?

Because management for better value requires tight control of innovation.

WHO?

The person who holds the money, the clinician making the bid, and the person who manages their resources.

WHEN?

This can be done as part of the annual planning process or as new technologies emerge.

HOW?

- The team that wants the new service should be asked to provide information about both the evidence-base and the relative value of the proposed innovation.

- The bid should be based on a systematic review of the evidence.

- The bidder should be required to prepare a systematic review if one is not available. If the evidence-base is inadequate, the bidder can be encouraged to bid for research funds.

- The bidder should provide data about:

  - The number of patients in the group or population they service who would be helped and harmed by the new service.

  - How the added benefits from the innovation compare with the added benefits that would result if the existing service were delivered at higher levels of quality.

- The relative value should be appraised, by asking the bidder to compare the value of this proposed addition to their service with:

  - Other innovations that the service might introduce in the next year.

  - The lowest value priority service they currently provide.

  - The problems that patients would face if some other part of the service were cut to fund this new service.

HOW TO CONDUCT AN ANNUAL POPULATION VALUE REVIEW

WHY?

To ensure that resources are allocated between different budgets to maximise value and identify the need for movement of resources from one budget to another.

WHO?

People responsible for allocation of resources.

WHEN?

In the middle of the financial year, when expenditure for the previous year is clear and expenditure for the next financial year is being planned.

HOW?

- Use a simple system of classification such as the International Classification of Diseases (ICD).

- Separate research and education costs.

- Allocate all other costs to the programme budgets, including primary care, laboratory and imaging.

- Distribute the budget analysis.

- Respond to criticisms by asking for suggestions about how allocation can be improved, but also by reminding people that it is their data and any quality problems start with them!

- For each budget, payers and managers should ask:

- What would be the effect on the value derived from resources if we:

  ○ increased the allocation to this programme by 5%?

  ○ decreased the allocation to this budget by 5%?

- Produce a report of these discussions and a proposal for reallocation of resources for the next financial year.

HOW TO CONDUCT A REVIEW OF EXPENDITURE ON A DISEASE

WHY?

Because the main focus of healthcare management, competition, and value improvement, should be on diseases, such as breast cancer, not on hospitals or insurance schemes.

WHO?

All those involved in managing resources for a particular condition, patients' representatives, and payers.

WHEN?

Because this activity requires energy and focus, and since there are about fifty 'big' problems such as epilepsy or diabetes, plan one a week throughout the year.

HOW

- Produce a value review pack containing data on
  - Hospital admissions compared with other services.
  - Prescribing rates compared with other services.
  - Outcome data, if available.
  - Any other data on variations in the care provided, from audit studies, for example.
  - Financial data, if available.
  - New high quality evidence produced in the preceding year.
- Present the pack to a Workshop.
- Accept criticisms of the data, reminding participants that 'These are the data you submitted.'
- Ask the Workshop to focus on their existing resources and ask:
  - What should we do more of, or better?
  - What should we do less?
- Ask the Workshop to advise:
  - What would be their top priority if new money became available?
  - What would be their lowest priority if cuts had to be made?
- Produce a value improvement plan.

HOW TO MANAGE KNOWLEDGE

WHY?

Because the implementation of what we know from research, from data, and from experience will have a bigger impact on health and healthcare than any other drug or technology likely to be developed in the next decade.

WHO?

The Chief Executive, Boards and Management Teams.

WHEN?

The management of knowledge needs to be reported to Executive Boards and Management Teams as frequently as financial reports.

HOW?

- The Chief Executive should identify one Board Member as responsible for knowledge and give that person the responsibility of being the Chief Knowledge Officer (CKO).

- Require the CKO to prepare a plan, describing how:

  ○ The knowledge coming into the organisation can be improved.

  ○ More knowledge from experience can be created within the organisation.

  ○ Important new knowledge can be more effectively implemented.

  ○ The knowledge produced by the organisation, e.g. patient leaflets, can be improved.

- Each significant management team in the organisation should also have one person on that team responsible for getting knowledge into practice.

- A librarian should be free from library management duties to support the CKO.

- Implement the plan.

HOW TO MANAGE INNOVATION

WHY?

Because organisations and individuals often adopt low value interventions while failing to develop or introduce high value interventions, unless innovation is managed.

WHO?

Every healthcare organisation that has a budget should have an Innovation Group, supported by the Chief Knowledge Officer and a librarian.

WHEN?

The group should meet regularly and produce an Annual Report.

HOW?

- Write a remit for the Innovation Group emphasising that:
  - its primary remit is to promote the development of new ways of working and to introduce new high value ideas from elsewhere;
  - its second priority is to promote research and evaluation and ensure that new services or interventions of uncertain value are introduced only in the context of research;
  - its third priority is to ensure that interventions of low value, new tests, new treatments, or new services are not introduced.
- Appoint an influential clinician as the Chair.
- Provide some resources to fund evaluations and encourage evaluators to publish their results.
- Ask the Chief Knowledge Officer and librarian to provide support to the group.
- Give the group one or two innovations that will be introduced on their recommendation in the first year.
- Support innovation schemes with rewards for teams who innovate to produce better value.
- Present an Annual Innovation Report to the Board.

HOW TO DO A SYSTEMATIC REVIEW

WHY?
A systematic review of all the evidence is necessary to minimise bias and errors in reports of research.

WHO?
The scale of a systematic review, and the skills required, should not be underestimated. Those who pay for or manage healthcare should commission someone who has experience to do the review.

WHEN?
Before significant resources are invested.

HOW?

- Make the question as precise as possible – e.g. instead of asking for a systematic review of PET scanners, ask 'What is the added value of PET scanning for patients with advanced cancer?'.

- Search the scientific literature with the assistance of a librarian and keep a copy of the search strategy.

- Use explicit quality criteria to decide which research reports should be included in the review and which should be excluded.

- Ask a statistician how the data in the individual high quality research reports should be combined.

- Publish the results of the review, including the references to the reports that were excluded for reasons of quality as well as the references that reports included in the review.

HOW TO REDUCE THE NUMBER OF ERRORS

WHY?

Because errors cause harm to patients, and costs to healthcare.

WHEN?

This needs to be a continuous process, but should have both an annual cycle, and specific actions as serious errors are identified.

WHO?

This needs to be a responsibility of every person who manages resources.

HOW?

- Promote continuous quality improvement, because improvement in quality will reduce the incidence of errors.

- Ask the Chief Knowledge Officer to review the knowledge about the types of errors likely to occur, and the evidence about the interventions which reduce risk.

- Set up a Risk Reduction Group, with a clearly accountable leader.

- Ask the group to develop and implement a risk reduction plan.

- Ensure there is a clear protocol for the investigation of errors, and the method by which patients can be involved in resolving problems caused by errors.

HOW TO ENGAGE PATIENTS AND IMPROVE THEIR EXPERIENCE

WHY?
Because the engagement of patients will improve the value of healthcare.

WHEN?
This is a continuous process, part of general management, but an annual patient engagement conference can highlight and focus this process.

WHO?
Every person who manages resources needs to be given this as a clear responsibility.

HOW?

- A person who can speak as a patient should be enrolled on the Board or management team.

- Review and improve complaint management.

- Reduce resources used in measuring patient satisfaction, and increase resources used to measure patient experience.

- Either develop your own patient experience questionnaire, using questions from sources such as www.healthcarecommission.com or commission an agency to conduct the surveys.

- Promote the use of the Database of Individual Patient Experience (www.dipex.org).

- Review the written information given to patients, and assure and improve the quality, using a tool such as DISCERN (www.discern.org).

- Ensure managers conduct experience surveys at least once a year and act on results; high quality surveys done for a short period are better value than continuous poor quality surveys.

HOW TO IMPROVE PRODUCTIVITY

WHY?
Because increased productivity frees resources for high value healthcare without adverse effects.

WHEN?
Continuously, obsessionally, but highlighted by an Annual Productivity Workshop and celebrations.

WHO?
Every person who manages resources. A Productivity Interest Group (PIG) to generate and support ideas can pull together leads from all the divisions (PIGs are very productive creatures!)

HOW?
- Ensure that everyone is clear about the distinction between efficiency and productivity, and that productivity does not mean a reduction in quality but an improvement in value.

- Develop and implement a communication plan.

- Set up projects to:
  - Make more use of buildings and equipment.
  - Improve procurement.
  - Reduce stock.
  - Launch a hospital-at-home project.
  - Reduce the use of paper.
  - Prevent the waste of resources on poor value research.
  - Make better use of the time of the most experienced staff.

- Require an Annual Productivity Report.

HOW TO INCREASE EFFECTIVENESS

WHY?
Because increased effectiveness increases value.

WHO?
Clinical leaders, including imaging, pharmacy and laboratory, and all people who manage resources.

WHEN?
Continuous process, built into annual planning and reporting, of the same status as finance.

HOW?

• Set up an Innovation Group to ensure that no ineffective technology slips into use.

• Require the Chief Knowledge Officer to produce monthly knowledge briefings about new evidence that should be put into practice.

• Develop systems of care, with care pathways for all common procedures and conditions, using software such as the Map of Medicine (www.mapofmedicine.com).

• For each condition, ask the relevant clinical lead to identify evidence-based measures of process and outcome measures of relevance to patients.

• Require each service to produce an Annual Effectiveness Plan, based on the annual review of their service and care.

• Require all Annual Reports to describe effectiveness compared with performance of other services and explicit national standards.

• Introduce the methods of continues quality improvement.

HOW TO GET TO THE ROOT OF PROBLEMS

WHY?

Because short-term solutions to immediate causes are of lower value than solutions which tackle root causes.

WHO?

Whoever has a problem.

WHEN?

Whenever there is a problem or an opportunity for value improvement that 'can't be done'.

HOW?

Use the Five Whys method of Taiichi Ohno, who always asked 'Why?' five times, for example:

Why is this patient at the clinic?	Because we have the reports of his investigations.
Why could the results not be sent to him?	Because a clinical decision needs to be made.
Why could he not make that decision with his primary care physician?	Because the physician does not know how we manage this problem.
Why does she not know how this problem is managed? Is it too difficult?	No it is not too difficult, but she is new to the area and not familiar with how we do things.
Why do we not identify and brief new GPs about our procedures?	'Good question'

HOW TO TRANSFORM HEALTHCARE USING INFORMATION TECHNOLOGY

WHY?

There are two reasons. Firstly, because the technology creates tools that by themselves change culture and practice – reflect on the lessons of history as described by Lynn White Jnr in *Medieval Technology and Social Change*. Secondly, because investing in Information Technology simply to do the same things digitally is of very low value – reflect on the lessons of 'How New Technologies Cause Great Companies To Fail' in *The Innovator's Dilemma* by Clayton Christensen.

WHO?

Everyone must be involved, but someone needs to take the lead in 'The Transformation of Care' not a project called 'The Introduction of IT'

WHEN?

Before every investment in IT.

HOW?

- Send the patient information digitally, linked to email if they have it, on a DVD if they do not, before and after every consultation.
- Encourage patients to record the consultation on their mobile phones.
- Offer email consultations.
- Train clinicians how to consult well with a computer in the consulting room.
- Describe all care pathways and standard operating procedures digitally, using the Map of Medicine software (www.medictomedic.com).
- Use IT to help multi-disciplinary teams work smarter.
- Make all knowledge available online.
- Create clinical networks which are sustained on the web, not by a bureaucracy.
- Put laboratory IT in charge of chronic disease monitoring.
- Get the Chief Executive to create a Blog.

PART IV

THE ETERNAL NEED FOR GOOD JUDGEMENT

In his classic study *Administrative Behaviour*, the fourth edition of which was published 50 years after the first, Nobel Prize winner Herbert Simon reflects on the interplay between ethical and factual decision-making and taking. He emphasises that 'the separation between the ethical and factual elements in judgement can usually be carried only a short distance.' (1) In theory, the bureaucrats or administrators make the decision by presenting facts, and the legislators or public representatives add the values, and take the final decision. 'Officials advise, Ministers decide' is the British maxim.

The advice of officials influences the decision-takers, and both can be influenced by expert advisers, usually scientists and doctors, not only by the strength of the evidence but also by the way it is expressed. One study found that the bureaucrats and legislators made different decisions if the same data were presented in different ways. (2) The interplay between expert, bureaucrat, and legislator is best analysed not in studies of healthcare but in the military context in *Winning The Next War*, an analysis of innovation, and opposition to innovation, in war and peace. (3)

The judgement of the payers is one which has to achieve a balance between the ideal economic option and the populist option, that which will satisfy most people. Every decision is taken as an ethical decision because every decision means that some group of patients will benefit and that others will suffer. The most commonly used ethical principle for decision-taking is probably 'utilitarianism' encapsulated into the phrase 'the greatest good for the greatest number', which sounds irresistible and is very popular.

However, the challenge to utilitarianism should always be borne in mind, as expressed by Dostoyevsky in *The Brothers Karamazov,* when Ivan asks Aloysha:

> '*Imagine that you are creating a fabric of human destiny with the object of making men happy in the end, giving them*

96

> *peace and rest at last, but that it was essential and inevitable*
> *to torture to death only one tiny creature – that baby beating*
> *its breast with its fist, for instance – and to found that edifice*
> *on its unavenged tears, would you consent to be the architect*
> *on those conditions?'*

Decision-takers may want to ensure both that they do the greatest good to the greatest number, and that they do the least harm to the smallest number. The high cost of treatment for people with rare diseases – high because there will never be a mass market for the 'orphan drugs' for treating rare conditions such as Gaucher's disease, for example – will increasingly challenge the values of decision-takers, as treatments for rare diseases become more common.

The need for 'Bounded Rationality'

Decision-taking is also an emotional business, leading Herbert Simon to describe the process as an example of 'Bounded Rationality'. Facts make a contribution, but only a contribution. Someone has to be responsible for taking decisions about resource allocation. Everyone wants to be part of decisions which allocate more resources; few people want to be part of decisions which cut allocations, or deny resources to groups of patients in need. But some poor devil has to do the job.

References

(1) Simon, H. (1997) Administrative Behaviour: A Study of Decision-Making Processes in Administrative Decisions. *Simon & Schuster*
(2) Fahey, T. et al (1995) Evidence-Based Purchasing. *BMJ 311: 1056-1060*
(3) Rosen, S.P. (1991) Winning the Next War: Innovation and the Modern Military. *Cornell University Press*

Index